EYE AND VISION RESEARCH DEVELOPMENTS

EYE DISEASES ASSOCIATED WITH SLEEP DISORDERS

EYE AND VISION RESEARCH DEVELOPMENTS

Additional books in this series can be found on Nova's website under the Series tab.

Additional e-books in this series can be found on Nova's website under the e-book tab.

EYE AND VISION RESEARCH DEVELOPMENTS

EYE DISEASES ASSOCIATED WITH SLEEP DISORDERS

MINGWU WANG, MD, PHD
EDITOR

NOVA BIOMEDICAL

New York

Library of Congress Cataloging-in-Publication Data

ISBN: 978-1-63482-894-9
Library of Congress Control Number: 2015939637

Published by Nova Science Publishers, Inc. † New York

Contents

Foreword

Joseph M. Miller, MD, MPH
The Murray and Clara Walker Chair of Ophthalmology
University of Arizona, Tucson, AZ, US

As a new resident in ophthalmology, I dreamed of sleep Finishing an internship before the intervention of "duty hours" for residents, [1] along with an infant at home, I imagined a quiet night-life of an ophthalmology resident. In-house call, a private room, no pesky baby noises at home—what a life!—only to discover that documenting "the diurnal curve" was an on-call responsibility. My first discovery of how sleep disturbance is associated with eye diseases was my own sleep disturbance in relation to the patient's glaucoma!

The diurnal variation of intraocular pressure was first described by Maslenikow in 1904. [2] Duke-Elder [3] then Drance [4] greatly contributed to the study of the biochemistry and endocrinology of sleep disorders through these early studies of diurnal variation in patients with glaucoma. The development of sleep medicine [5] and the recognition of the multitude of interactions sleep disorders with health have led to an explosion of understanding of the biology of diurnal variation, sleep, and dark rest. We now know that sleep is more than a luxury, it is a biological necessity, and that sleep disturbance results in more than a grumpy doctor – it interferes with homeostasis. If rats are kept awake for two weeks, they become hypermetabolic, lose homeostatic function, and die. [6]

This book brings together a collection of chapters that summarize recognized interactions of sleep health with eye health.

Beginning with a case presentation and providing the non-ophthalmologists with a brief background of the eye disease, each chapter then moves into the literature associating the pathophysiology of sleep disorders with the respective eye disorder.

Mingwu Wang MD, PhD, the lead author of this text, has recruited an outstanding group of contributors of these clinical vignettes from fellow faculty and resident physicians of the University of Arizona. He has drawn on the expertise of colleagues across the breadth of Ophthalmology to summarize the current state of knowledge of sleep disorder associated eye diseases

Anterior manifestations of sleep disorder associated eye findings include disorders of the eyelid, ocular surface, and degenerative corneal changes. Dry eye disease is perhaps the most commonly experienced sleep deprivation associated eye finding, is covered in its own chapter by Duncan and Wang. Sobti et al. summarize the association between floppy eyelid syndrome and obstructive sleep apnea (OSA), well known but commonly under recognized clinical entities. Stevenson and Wang cover the available evidence linking keratoconus (a leading indication for corneal transplant) and OSA.

The impact of sleep disorders on optic nerve, on the other hand, is much more vision threatening. Glaucoma has been recognized as a complex disease representing an optic neuropathy of which intraocular pressure is but one risk factor. Choo and Tsai presented evidence of the contribution of sleep disorders to the development of glaucoma, a truly complex topic. Nonarteritic anterior ischemic optic neuropathy (NAION), frequently presents as abrupt vision loss on awakening in the morning, has provoked tremendous research in the association of OSA and NAION. Altenbernd and Smith describe the evidence base for such an association. Papilledema, optic nerve swelling as a result of elevated intracranial pressure, represents an ocular manifestation of disorders in the central nervous system. Cho and Yu analyzed accumulated data suggesting the role of abnormal sleep as an etiology of papilledema in a separate topic.

Last but not least, Christoforidis and others describe the association between sleep disorders and three important retinal diseases: diabetic retinopathy, retinal vein occlusion and central serous chorioretinopathy. The mounting evidence of retinal diseases attributable to sleep disorders is ever intriguing.

Rechtshaffen, in his seminal investigations on the association of sleep deprivation on the health of rats, notes that seeing what happens when a vital function (sleep) is blocked is not the same as knowing what ***is*** the function of sleep itself. Perhaps, just as the discovery of rapid eye movement (REM) sleep inaugurated the science of sleep, there are further advances to be had by investigating the relation of the eye and sleep. We hope that this text may help you open your eyes to what may happen when your eyes are closed.

References

[1] Resident Duty Hours: Enhancing Sleep, Supervision, and Safety: Cheryl Ulmer, Dianne Miller Wolman, Michael M.E. Johns, Editors, Committee on Optimizing Graduate Medical Trainee (Resident) Hours and Work Schedule to Improve Patient Safety, National Research Council National Academy Press, Washington DC, 2009. Available for download at www.nap.edu.

[2] Maslenikow A: Uber Tagesschwankungen des intraokularen Druckesbei Glaukom, Z Augenheilk 11:564, 1904.

[3] Duke-Elder S: The Phasic Variations in the Ocular Tension in Primary Glaucoma. *Am J Ophthal* 35(1):1-21, 1952.

[4] Drance, S. M: The Significance of the Diurnal Tension Variations in Normal and Glaucomatous Eyes, *Arch Ophthal* 64:494-501, 1960.

[5] Shepard JW, Buysse DJ, Chesson AL, et al: History of the Development of Sleep Medicine in the United States *J Clin Sleep Med.* 1(1): 61–82, 2005 Jan.

[6] Rechtschaffen A, Bergmann BM: Sleep deprivation in the rat: an update of the 1989 Paper. *Sleep.* 1;25(1):18-24, 2002 Feb.

In: Eye Diseases …
Editor: Mingwu Wang
ISBN: 978-1-63482-894-9

Chapter 1

Sleep Disorders and Neuroregulation

Hong Lei[1]*, MD, PhD and Mingwu Wang[2], MD, PhD
[1]Department of Neurology,
[2]Departments of Ophthalmology and Vision Science,
University of Arizona College of Medicine, AZ, US

Sleep disorders are extremely common in the general population, with reports that up to 30 percent of the population experience sleep disturbances lasting at least several nights per month. [1] Sleep disorders may cause or exacerbate preexisting medical and psychiatric conditions and are associated with high rates of depression, anxiety, and impaired daytime functioning. [2] They may also lead to poor occupational performance, motor vehicle accidents, cardiovascular and endocrine disorders, heightened pain perception, and ocular diseases. [3, 4] This chapter provides an introduction to sleep disorders and their connections with neuroregulation, and discusses possible links between sleep disorders and ocular diseases.

* E-mail: leih@email.arizona.edu.

1. Normal Sleep

According to a simple behavioral definition, *sleep* is a reversible behavioral state of perceptual disengagement from and unresponsiveness to the environment, [5] and is usually associated with a species-specific sleep posture, selection of location, and circadian timing. The occurrence of sleep has been inferred on the basis of a variety of criteria that range from simple observation of posture, behavior, and/or eye state to almost complete reliance on the electroencephalogram (EEG) in sleep studies. For clinical and experimental purposes, vigilance states and stages of sleep are defined principally on the basis of characteristic patterns of the EEG, eye movement as detected by electrooculogram (EOG), and muscle tone measured by electromyogram (EMG). This collection of such records is known as a polysomnogram (PSG). Polysomnographic profiles define three distinct states of vigilance: wakefulness, nonrapid-eye-movement sleep (NREMS), and rapid-eye-movement sleep (REMS).

Each of these three sleep states has different physiologic controls and functions. Additionally, NREMS can be further subdivided into four stages. [5] Stage 1 sleep marks the transition from waking to sleep. This stage is characterized by slowing of the EEG frequency, reduction in muscle tone, and low arousal threshold. Stage 2 sleep is characterized by the occurrence of sleep spindles (7- to 14-Hz bursts that reflect thalamocortical synchronization), K complexes (large biphasic waves with ultralow rhythm that reflect initial cortical synchronization), a higher arousal threshold, and, as stage 2 progresses, the gradual appearance of high-amplitude slow waves in the EEG. Sleep stages 3 and 4 are characterized by a predominance of high-amplitude signals in the slow-frequency (delta frequency band, or < 4-Hz) component of the EEG, and hence are often called slow-wave sleep (SWS) or delta sleep. As the result of a modification of standard guidelines by the American Academy of Sleep Medicine in 2008, the category of NREM stage 4 sleep has been eliminated; consequently, stages 3 and 4 are now considered to be a single stage labeled as stage 3.

Whereas NREM sleep, which is dreamless and accounts for 75-80 percent of sleep time in an adult human, REM sleep is typically associated with dreaming and accounts for 20-25 percent of total sleep time. REM sleep has tonic and phasic components; in addition the length of the REM period and density of eye movements increase throughout the sleep cycle. [6] REM sleep follows NREM sleep and occurs 4-5 times during a normal 8-hour sleep period. The first REM period of the night may be less than 10 minutes in duration, while the last may exceed 60 minutes. The NREM-REM cycles vary in length from 70-100 minutes initially to 90-120 minutes later in the night. Typically, Stage 3 sleep occurs more frequently in the first third of the night, whereas REM sleep predominates in the last third of the night. Awareness of this pattern can be helpful clinically as NREM parasomnias such as sleepwalking typically occur in the first third of the night with the presence of Stage 3 sleep. This contrasts with REM sleep behavior disorder (RBD), which typically occurs in the last half of the night.

2. Neuroregulation of Normal Sleep

The concept that sleep and waking are controlled by some chemical changes has evolved over time. Historically, sleep was thought to be a passive state that was initiated through withdrawal of sensory input. Currently, withdrawal of sensory awareness is believed to be a factor in sleep since an active initiation mechanism that facilitates brain withdrawal has been recognized. [7] It is now believed that the process of sleep is regulated by interactions of multiple anatomic and neurochemical processes within the central nervous system. Both homeostatic factors and circadian factors interact to determine the timing and quality of sleep.

The origin of sleep is considered to reside in the ventrolateral preoptic nucleus (VLPO) of the anterior hypothalamus. This area becomes active during sleep and uses the neurotransmitters GABA and galanin, which initiate sleep by inhibiting the arousal regions of the brain The VLPO innervates and can inhibit the wake-promoting regions of the brain including the tuberomammillary nucleus, lateral hypothalamus, locus coeruleus, dorsal raphe, laterodorsal tegmental nucleus, and pedunculopontine tegmental (PPT) nucleus. The hypocretin (orexin) neurons in the lateral hypothalamus help stabilize this switch. Significantly, when the hypocretin neurons are lost, narcolepsy can result. [8]

Inhibition of the tuberoinfundibular region, which projects rostrally to the intralaminar nuclei of the thalamus and then to the cerebral cortex, is a critical step toward falling asleep because it results in functional disconnection between the brain stem and the more rostral thalamus and cortex. A decrease in ascending thalamic cholinergic transmissions occurs in association with decreasing cortical responsiveness In addition to inhibiting higher cortical consciousness, the tuberoinfundibular tract, which projects caudally into the pontine reticular system, inhibits afferent transmissions from ascending cholinergic tracts. [9]

The suprachiasmatic nucleus, located in the hypothalamus, serves as a pacemaker, responsible for generating the circadian rhythm The pineal gland secretes less melatonin when exposed to bright light; therefore, the level of this chemical is lowest during the daytime hours of wakefulness. It has become increasingly clear that rhythms in metabolic processes are not simply responses to daily environmental/behavioral influences, but are also driven in part by cell autonomous circadian clocks. By synchronizing the cells with their environment, these clocks modulate a host of metabolic processes in a temporally appropriate manner. [10]

There are a wide variety of compounds which are thought to have neuroregulatory properties, either as neurotransmitters or as modulators of neuronal function. [11] These include serotonin from the dorsal raphe nucleus, norepinephrine contained in neurons with cell bodies in the locus ceruleus, and acetylcholine from the pontine reticular formation Dopamine, on the other hand, is associated with wakefulness. Abnormalities in the delicate balance of all of these chemical messenger systems may disrupt various physiologic, biologic, behavioral, and EEG parameters responsible for REM sleep and NREM sleep.

NREM is an active state that is maintained partly through oscillations between the thalamus and the cortex Sleep spindles, a hallmark of stage 2 sleep, are generated by bursts of hyperpolarizing GABAnergic neurons in the reticular nucleus of the thalamus. These bursts inhibit thalamocortical projection neurons. As deafferentation spreads, corticothalamic projections, which extend back to the thalamus, synchronize As hyperpolarization of the thalamic reticular neurons progresses, delta waves are produced by interactions from both thalamic reticular and cortical pyramidal sources. Slow cortical oscillations are produced in neocortical networks by cyclic hyperpolarizations and depolarizations. Although the functions of NREM sleep remain speculative, several theories have been put forth. One theory proposes that decreased metabolic demand facilitates replenishment of glycogen stores. Another theory, which utilizes neuronal plasticity, suggests that the oscillating depolarizations and hyperpolarizations consolidate memory and remove redundant or excess synapses. [12]

REM sleep is generated by the cholinergic mediated “REM-on neurons” in the mesencephalic and pontine cholinergic neurons. The PPT nucleus and the lateral dorsal tegmental (LDT) neurons use acetylcholine to trigger cortical desynchrony via the thalamus Cortical desynchrony (also described as low voltage mixed frequency) is the EEG hallmark of REM sleep. An additional EEG hallmark of REM sleep is "sawtooth waves." A pharmacologic offshoot of the cholinergic mediation is that REM sleep increases with cholinergic agonists and decreases with anticholinergics. "REM-off neurons" are the monoadrenergic locus ceruleus and serotonergic raphe neurons. The REM-off neurons use norepinephrine, serotonin, and histamine to inhibit the REM-on cholinergic cells and stop REM sleep. These REM-off neurons become inactive during REM sleep. Notably, medications such as antidepressants, that increase the amount of norepinephrine or serotonin can cause a pharmacologic suppression of REM sleep. [9, 13]

Projection of the presumed cholinergic, dorsolateral, small-cell, reticular group occurs through the medullary reticular formation, which projects through the ventrolateral reticulospinal tract to inhibitory spinal and bulbar interneurons. Glycinergic interneurons produce postsynaptic inhibition and hyperpolarization of the spinal alpha motor neurons. Tonic cortical activation with EEG desynchronization is promoted by projections from cholinergic lateral dorsal tegmental and pedunculopontine tegmental neurons to the thalamic nuclei. Other projections through brainstem reticular formation neurons are likely to be involved as well.

As noted earlier, REM sleep is characterized by muscle atonia, cortical activation, low-voltage desynchronization of the EEG, and rapid eye movements. [14] REM sleep has a parasympathetically mediated tonic component and a sympathetically mediated phasic component. The phasic portion of REM sleep is characterized by skeletal muscle twitches, increased heart rate variability, pupil dilation, and increased respiratory rate. [15] Muscle atonia, which is present throughout REM sleep except for phasic muscle twitches, results from inhibition of alpha motor neurons by clusters of peri–locus ceruleus neurons, which are referred to collectively as the dorsolateral small cell reticular group. Phasic rapid eye movements are composed of lateral saccades generated in the paramedian pontine reticular formation and vertical saccades, which are thought to be generated in the mesencephalic reticular formation. REM density is a term used to describe the frequency per minute of the eye movement bursts.

During NREM sleep, the metabolic demand of the brain decreases. This is supported by oxygen positron emission tomography (PET) studies, which show that during NREM sleep the blood flow throughout the entire brain progressively decreases. PET studies also show that during REM sleep blood flow increases in the thalamus and the primary visual, motor, and sensory cortices, while remaining comparatively decreased in the prefrontal and parietal associational regions. The increase in blood flow to the primary visual regions of the cortex may explain the vivid nature of REM dreaming, while the continued decrease in blood flow to the prefrontal cortex may explain the unquestioning acceptance of even the most bizarre dream content. [16, 17]

3. Abnormal Sleep

I. Classification of Sleep Disorders

Sleep disorders may be primary or secondary, stemming from a variety of psychiatric and medical conditions. Primary sleep disorders result from an endogenous disturbance in the sleep-wake generating or timing mechanism often complicated by behavioral conditioning They may be divided into the following two broad categories. *Dyssomnias* are characterized by abnormalities in the amount, quality, or timing of sleep; they include primary insomnia and hypersomnia, narcolepsy, breathing-related sleep disorder such as sleep apnea, and circadian rhythm sleep disorder. *Parasomnias* are unusual experiences or behaviors that occur during sleep; they include sleep terror disorder, restless leg syndrome (RLS), sleepwalking, and nightmare disorder.

II. Clinical Approach

a) Sleep History

A sleep history should include bedtime habits, timing of sleep onset and waking, daytime sleepiness, snoring, abnormal nocturnal leg kicking, nocturia, mood complaints, and cataplexy Details about comorbid medical or psychiatric diagnoses, substance abuse, stressors, and family history should also be elicited. A daily sleep log and the Epworth Sleepiness Scale (ESS) [18] can be utilized for gathering information.

b) Specific Physical Examination

An evaluation for obstructive sleep apnea (OSA) should include measurements of neck circumference and posterior airway size. Neck circumferences greater than 43 cm in men or 41 cm in women are associated with increased OSA risk The Mallampati classification, which assigns a score to grade the severity of airway crowding, and a higher score together with nasal obstruction, rates risk factors for OSA. RLS may be associated with peripheral neuropathy, and in these patients, a careful sensory examination of the lower extremities is indicated. Similarly, RBD may be a harbinger for alpha synucleinopathies, such as Parkinson disease, which may become apparent on clinical evaluation and is associated with nocturnal agitation and dream enactment. [19]

c) Objective Tests

Although many sleep disorders can be diagnosed clinically, some require further evaluation in a sleep laboratory. In suspected sleep-related breathing disorders, a full night PSG is recommended followed by continuous positive airway pressure (CPAP) titration. Home testing with a portable monitoring (PM) has become another acceptable form of objective testing. [20] A PSG is also indicated in severe forms of parasomnias, such as RBD. Patients who have possible narcolepsy should be evaluated with a multiple sleep latency test (MSLT) for objective quantification of hypersomnia, and a PSG performed the night before to document total sleep time to evaluate for other comorbid sleep disturbances.

Alternatively, insomnia and RLS do not routinely require a PSG because diagnosis is mainly clinically derived. [6] In some circumstances, a PSG may be helpful for some who present with insomnia that is refractory to traditional therapy and in whom other sleep disorders (e.g., sleep apnea, motor disorders of sleep) are also suspected. The indices commonly used to assess sleep disordered breathing (SDB) are the apnea-hypopnea index (AHI) and the respiratory disturbance index (RDI) The AHI is defined as the average number of episodes of apnea and hypopnea per hour. The RDI is defined as the average number of respiratory disturbances (obstructive apneas, hypopneas, and respiratory event–related arousals [RERAs]) per hour.

4. Common Sleep Disorders

Insomnia may present as decreased sleep efficiency or decreased total hours of sleep, with some associated decrease in productivity or well-being Because sleep requirements vary from person to person, the quality of sleep is more important than the total number of hours slept.

Initial insomnia (also referred to as early insomnia or sleep-onset insomnia) is characterized by difficulty in falling asleep, with an increase in sleep latency (i.e., the time between going to bed and falling asleep). Initial insomnia is frequently related to anxiety disorder s. Middle insomnia (also referred to as sleep-maintenance insomnia) refers to difficulty in maintaining sleep. Decreased sleep efficiency is present, with fragmented unrestful sleep and frequent waking during the night. Middle insomnia may be associated with medical illness, pain syndromes, or depression In terminal insomnia (also referred to as late insomnia or early morning wakening insomnia), patients consistently wake up earlier than needed. This symptom is frequently associated with major depression Alterations of the sleep-wake cycle may be a sign of circadian rhythm disturbances, such as those caused by jet lag and shift work.

Hypersomnia, or *excessive daytime sleepiness,* is characterized by recurrent episodes of excessive daytime sleepiness or prolonged nighttime sleep that has occurred for at least three months prior to diagnosis. [21] As opposed to feeling tired due to lack of sleep or interrupted sleep at night, persons with hypersomnia are compelled to nap repeatedly during the day, often at inappropriate times such as at work, driving, or in conversation. These daytime naps usually provide no relief from symptoms. Hypersomnia may be caused by other sleep disorders (such as narcolepsy, sleep apnea), dysfunction of the autonomic nervous system, or drug or alcohol abuse. In some cases, it results from medical conditions such as head trauma, depression, malignancy, or obesity. Some people appear to have a genetic predisposition to hypersomnia; in others, there is no known cause.

Obstructive sleep apnea is characterized by repeated episodes of a decrease or complete halt in airflow despite an ongoing effort to breathe. It occurs when the muscles relax during sleep, causing soft tissue in the back of the throat to collapse and block the upper airway. This leads to partial reductions (hypopneas) and complete pauses (apnea s) in breathing that last at least 10 seconds during sleep. Most pauses last between 10 and 30 seconds, but some may persist for one minute or longer. This can lead to abrupt reductions in blood oxygen saturation.

The brain responds to the lack of oxygen by alerting the body, causing a brief arousal from sleep that restores normal breathing This pattern can occur hundreds of times in one night. The result is a fragmented quality of sleep that often produces an excessive level of daytime sleepiness. Most people with OSA snore loudly and frequently, with periods of silence when airflow is reduced or blocked. They then make choking, snorting or gasping sounds when their airway reopens.

In adults, the diagnosis of OSA is confirmed when either of the two conditions exists: [22]

1) There are five or more predominantly obstructive respiratory events such as obstructive and mixed apnea s, hypopneas, or RERAs per hour of sleep for polysomnography or recording time for out of center sleep testing (OCST) in a patient with one or more of the following:
   - Sleepiness, nonrestorative sleep, fatigue, or insomnia symptoms;
   - Waking up with breath holding, gasping, or choking;
   - Habitual snoring, breathing interruptions, or both noted by a bed partner or other observer;
   - Hypertension, mood disorder, cognitive dysfunction, coronary artery disease, stroke, congestive heart failure, atrial fibrillation, or type 2 diabetes mellitus
2) There are fifteen or more predominantly obstructive respiratory events (apneas, hypopneas, or RERAs) per hour of sleep (for polysomnography) or recording time (for OCST), regardless of the presence of associated symptoms or comorbidities.

Whether the AHI or RDI should be the gold standard index remains unclear. Outcome studies are needed to determine which index should be preferred. The main implication of the difference is that the RDI classifies more patients as having OSA than does the AHI, using the same threshold values. In addition, most OCST devices do not include EEG monitoring, and therefore RERAs and hypopneas characterized by arousals cannot be identified. Although the AHI alone is not entirely predictive of the presence and severity of symptoms and complications, the following is a general description of patients in each category.

Mild: Patients who have an AHI between 5 and 15 respiratory events per hour of sleep Such patients may be relatively asymptomatic or report sedentary (e.g., passive) daytime sleepiness, becoming noticeable once the patient is unstimulated.

Moderate: Patients who have an AHI between 15 and 30 respiratory events per hour of sleep Such patients are typically aware of daytime sleepiness and take steps to avoid falling asleep at inappropriate times (e.g., taking a nap or avoiding driving long distances).

Severe: Patients who have an AHI greater than 30 respiratory events per hour of sleep and/or an oxyhemoglobin saturation below 90 percent for more than 20 percent of the total sleep time. Such patients more often have daytime sleepiness that interferes with normal daily activities.

Narcolepsy Diagnostic criteria include symptoms of severe excessive daytime sleepiness occurring almost daily for at least three months that interfere with functioning, REM intrusion phenomena (e.g., cataplexy, hypnagogic hallucinations, sleep paralysis), and electrographic evidence of an abnormal MSLT, with a sleep latency of 8 minutes or less and at least two sleep-onset REM periods following a PSG. Narcolepsy may occur with or without cataplexy.

Cataplexy is defined as sudden self-limited episodes of loss of waking muscle tone, usually triggered by laughter or other strong emotions. The presence of cataplexy may be sufficient by itself to establish the diagnosis of narcolepsy, although sleep studies are often advised to quantitatively assess the level of sleepiness. Sleep paralysis occurs as patients transition from sleep to waking, and consists of episodes up to several minutes in duration of inability to move and occasionally feeling unable to breathe despite being awake. Hypnagogic hallucinations are vivid and often frightening, which occur during the transition between waking and sleep. Sleep paralysis and hypnagogic hallucinations may rarely occur in normal individuals also.

Sleepwalking, also called *somnambulism*, involves episodes of complex behaviors including getting up and walking around while in a state of sleep These episodes occur during NREM sleep (stages 3 and 4), of which the patient is amnestic afterward. More common in children than adults, sleepwalking is usually outgrown by the teen years. Isolated incidents of sleepwalking do not often signal any serious problems or require treatment However, recurrent sleepwalking may suggest an underlying sleep disorder

Nightmares are repeated awakenings from sleep caused by vivid and distressing recall of dreams. Nightmares usually occur during the second half of the sleep period. Upon wakening from the dream, the person rapidly reorients to time and place.

Night terrors are recurrent episodes of abrupt awakening from sleep characterized by a panicky scream, with intense fear and autonomic arousal The individual usually has no recall of the details of the event and is unresponsive during the episode. Night terrors occur during the first third of the night, during stages 3 and 4 of NREM sleep.

Restless leg syndrome is characterized by uncomfortable sensations in the legs, especially when sitting or lying down, accompanied by an irresistible urge to move the affected limb. Symptoms occur primarily at night when a person is relaxing or at rest and can increase in severity during the night. Moving the legs relieves the discomfort Although the syndrome is idiopathic in most cases, RLS appears to be more common in patients with peripheral neuropathy, anemia and kidney failure In other cases, substances such as tricyclic antidepressants, caffeine, and antihistamines may be implicated. More than 80 percent of people with RLS also experience a more common condition known as periodic limb movement of sleep (PLMS). PLMS is characterized by involuntary leg twitching or jerking movements during sleep that typically occur every 15 to 40 seconds, sometimes throughout the night. The symptoms cause repeated awakening and severely disrupted sleep. Although many individuals with RLS also develop PLMS, most people with PLMS do not experience RLS. People who have PLMS and do not have RLS or another cause for the PLMS may be diagnosed with periodic limb movement disorder, which may be a variant of RLS.

There is no specific test for RLS. The four basic criteria for diagnosing the disorder are:

- Symptoms that are worse at night and are absent or negligible in the morning;
- A strong and often overwhelming need or urge to move the affected limb(s), often associated with paresthesias (abnormal sensations) or dysesthesias (unpleasant abnormal sensations);
- Sensory symptoms that are triggered by rest, relaxation, or sleep; and
- Sensory symptoms that are relieved with movement and the relief persists as long as the movement continues.

5. Impact of Sleep Disorders on Pathogenesis of Ocular Diseases

Although the physiopathology of sleep disorders and their links to ocular diseases are not yet fully understood, the effects of sleep disorders with changes in neuroregulation in relation to homeostasis provide insight into how such changes can play a role in the pathogenesis of ocular dysfunction. Ample correlations have been found in some sleep disorders such as OSA while connections with other sleep disorders require further investigation. Nevertheless, subjects with sleep disorders often share the disorders of the arousal system, with chronic activation (e.g., hyperarousal) of stress response, [23] increased metabolic rate, increased cortisol secretion, increased heart rate, and decreased heart rate variability. [24] Also, sleep loss as consequences of sleep disorders alters molecular processes that drive cellular immune activation and induce inflammatory cytokines. [25]

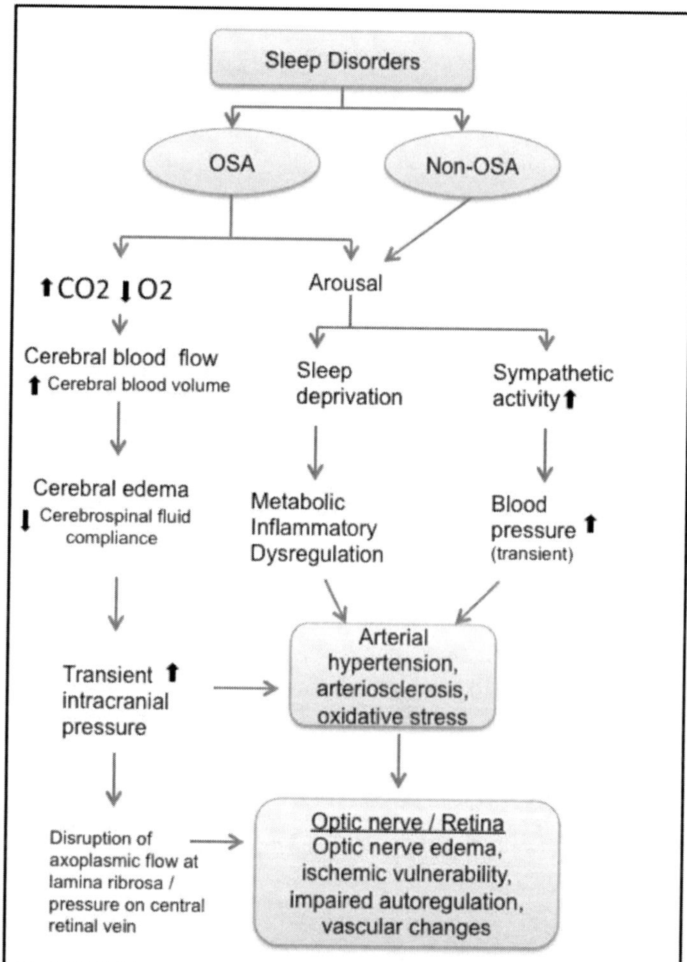

Figure 1. Physiologic effects of sleep disorders on homeostasis and the possible pathogenesis of ocular diseases OSA: obstructive sleep apnea

In summary, sleep disorders may contribute to ocular diseases through direct or indirect mechanisms (Figure 1). Among the mechanisms associated with sleep disorders, the following may be closely implicated in ocular diseases: intermittent sympathetic activity and sleep disturbance result in transient elevations in blood pressure and a number of hemodynamic changes. [26] Alterations in vascular functioning can lead to arteriosclerosis or impair the autoregulatory capacity of the optic nerve, leaving it vulnerable to ischemic events. [27] In addition, the immediate physiological effects of OSA involve hypoxia, hypercapnia, and inspiratory effort. These factors may directly impact the functioning of the optic nerve or work in concert to manifest as vascular sequelae. [28] Moreover, direct exposure to hypoxia and hypercapnia has been hypothesized to lead to damage of the optic nerve. Large fluctuations in vascular oxygen and carbon dioxide function as metabolic stresses that may overwhelm the autoregulatory capacity of the optic nerve head and retina. [29] Further, hypoxia-induced cerebral vasodilatation impedes cerebral perfusion pressure, [30] which may ultimately hinder autoregulation. Finally, decreased intrathoracic pressure created by inspiratory effort leads to increased venous return, [31] which can lead to elevation of the intraocular pressure.

The process of sleep is regulated by interactions of multiple anatomic and neurochemical processes within the central nervous system While much work remains to be done in elucidating the links between sleep disorders and ocular dysfunction, the study of sleep neuroregulation and homeostasis promises to increase our knowledge of mechanisms underlying ocular diseases.

Acknowledgment

Karen Wells, PhD, for her assistance with English editing.

References

[1] Thorpy M. J. Approach to the patient with a sleep complaint. *Semin. Neurol.*, 2004; 24:225-235.

[2] Breslau N., Roth T., Rosenthal L., Andreski P. Sleep disturbance and psychiatric disorders: a longitudinal epidemiological study of young adults *Biol. Psychiatry,* 1996; 39:411-418.

[3] Copinschi G. Metabolic and endocrine effects of sleep deprivation *Essent. Psychopharmacol.*, 2005; 6:341-347.

[4] Dhillon S., Shapiro C. M., Flanagan J. Sleep-disordered breathing and effects on ocular health *Can. J. Ophthalmol.,* 2007; 42:238-243.

[5] Kryger M. H., Roth T., Dement W. C. Principles and practice of sleep medicine, 4th ed. Philadelphia, PA: Elsevier/Saunders, 2005.

[6] Berry R. B., Budhiraja R., Gottlieb D. J., et al. Rules for scoring respiratory events in sleep: update of the 2007 AASM Manual for the Scoring of Sleep and Associated Events. Deliberations of the Sleep Apnea Definitions Task Force of the American Academy of Sleep Medicine. *J. Clin. Sleep Med.,* 2012; 8:597-619.

[7] Siegel J. M. Clues to the functions of mammalian sleep *Nature,* 2005; 437:1264-1271.

[8] Siegel J. M., Moore R., Thannickal T., Nienhuis R. A brief history of hypocretin/orexin and narcolepsy *Neuropsychopharmacology,* 2001; 25:S14-20.

[9] Espana R. A., Scammell T. E. Sleep neurobiology for the clinician. *Sleep,* 2004; 27:811-820.

[10] Bailey S. M., Udoh U. S., Young M. E. Circadian regulation of metabolism *J. Endocrinol.,* 2014; 222:R75-96.

[11] Holman R. B., Elliott G. R., Barchas J. D. Neuroregulators and sleep mechanisms. *Annu. Rev. Med.,* 1975; 26:499-520.

[12] Chokroverty S., ed. Physiologic changes in sleep Boston: Butterworth-Heinemann, 1999.

[13] Saper C. B., Scammell T. E., Lu J. Hypothalamic regulation of sleep and circadian rhythms *Nature,* 2005; 437:1257-1263.

[14] Morrison A. R. Coming to grips with a "new" state of consciousness: the study of rapid-eye-movement sleep in the 1960s. *J. Hist. Neurosci.,* 2013; 22:392-407.

[15] Tobaldini E., Nobili L., Strada S., Casali K. R., Braghiroli A., Montano N. Heart rate variability in normal and pathological sleep *Front. Physiol.*, 2013; 4:294.

[16] Desseilles M., Dang-Vu T., Schabus M., Sterpenich V., Maquet P., Schwartz S. Neuroimaging insights into the pathophysiology of sleep disorders *Sleep,* 2008; 31:777-794.

[17] Braun A. R., Balkin T. J., Wesenten N. J., et al. Regional cerebral blood flow throughout the sleep-wake cycle. An H2(15)O PET study. *Brain,* 1997; 120 (Pt 7):1173-1197.

[18] Johns M. W. A new method for measuring daytime sleepiness: the Epworth sleepiness scale. *Sleep,* 1991; 14:540-545.

[19] Boeve B. F., Silber M. H., Ferman T. J. REM sleep behavior disorder in Parkinson's disease and dementia with Lewy bodies. *J. Geriatr. Psychiatry Neurol.*, 2004; 17:146-157.

[20] Epstein L. J., Kristo D., Strollo P. J., Jr., et al. Clinical guideline for the evaluation, management and long-term care of obstructive sleep apnea in adults *J. Clin. Sleep Med.*, 2009; 5:263-276.

[21] Dauvilliers Y. Differential diagnosis in hypersomnia *Curr. Neurol. Neurosci. Rep.*, 2006; 6:156-162.

[22] International Classification of Sleep Disorders, 3rd ed. Darien, IL American Academy of Sleep Medicine, 2014.

[23] Elam M., Sverrisdottir Y. B., Rundqvist B., McKenzie D., Wallin B. G., Macefield V. G. Pathological sympathoexcitation: how is it achieved? *Acta Physiol. Scand.*, 2003; 177:405-411.

[24] Dowling T. C. Prevalence, etiology, and consequences of anemia and clinical and economic benefits of anemia correction in patients with chronic kidney disease: an overview. *Am. J. Health Syst. Pharm.,* 2007; 64:S3-7; quiz S23-25.

[25] Irwin M. R., Wang M., Campomayor C. O., Collado-Hidalgo A., Cole S. Sleep deprivation and activation of morning levels of cellular and genomic markers of inflammation *Arch. Intern. Med.*, 2006; 166:1756-1762.

[26] Bao X., Nelesen R. A., Loredo J. S., Dimsdale J. E., Ziegler M. G. Blood pressure variability in obstructive sleep apnea: role of sympathetic nervous activity and effect of continuous positive airway pressure *Blood Press Monit.*, 2002; 7:301-307.

[27] Hayreh S. S. Blood supply of the optic nerve head. *Ophthalmologica,* 1996; 210:285-295.

[28] Zgaga L., Hayward C., Vatavuk Z., et al. High prevalence of glaucoma in Veli Brgud, Croatia, is caused by a dominantly inherited T377M mutation in the MYOC gene. *Br. J. Ophthalmol.*, 2008; 92:1567-1568.

[29] Orgul S., Gugleta K., Flammer J. Physiology of perfusion as it relates to the optic nerve head. *Surv. Ophthalmol.,* 1999; 43 Suppl. 1:S17-26.

[30] Pearce W. J. Mechanisms of hypoxic cerebral vasodilatation. *Pharmacol. Ther.*, 1995; 65:75-91.

[31] Scharf S. M. The effect of decreased intrathoracic pressure on ventricular function. *J. Sleep Res.*, 1995; 4:53-58.

In: Eye Diseases …
Editor: Mingwu Wang

ISBN: 978-1-63482-894-9

Chapter 2

Floppy Eyelid Syndrome and Obstructive Sleep Apnea

Deepak Sobti[1]*, MD, Kamel Itani[1], MD, James Merritt[2], MD and Ronald Mancini[1], MD
[1]Department of Ophthalmology,
University of Texas Southwestern Medical Center,
[2]Oculoplastic Associates of Texas, TX, US

Case Presentation

A 46-year-old obese man with a history of dermatochalasis presents for an evaluation of foreign body sensation for several months in both eyes. At the last encounter, mild symptomatic improvement was obtained with artificial tears. On physical examination his eyelids demonstrate lower eyelid laxity and the upper eyelids are easily everted (Figure 1). Slit-lamp biomicroscopy reveals papillary conjunctivitis.

These findings prompted further evaluation with overnight polysomnography. A result of obstructive sleep apnea confirmed a diagnosis of floppy eyelid syndrome.

* E-mail: deepak.sobti.md@gmail.com.

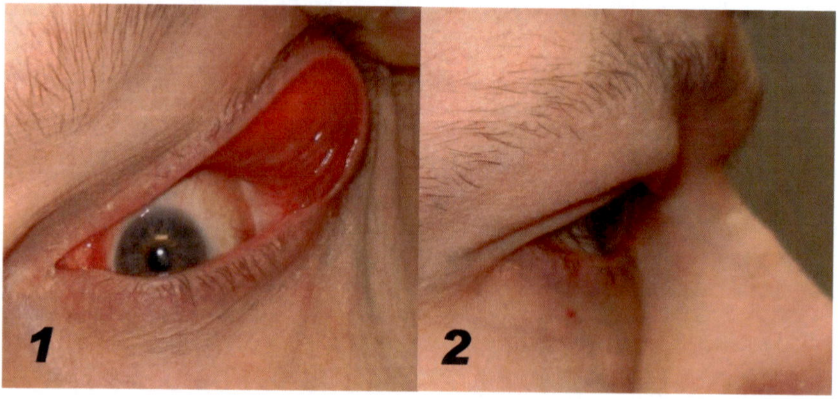

Color photographs taken of an obese male with floppy eyelid syndrome Figure 1. Note the marked laxity seen as easily everted eyelids with upward traction. Figure 2. Note the downward direction of eyelashes of the right upper eyelid known as eyelash ptosis (Photo courtesy: James Merritt, MD).

Floppy Eyelid Syndrome: An Overview

Floppy eyelid syndrome (FES) was first described by Culbertson and Ostler in 1981. [1] The authors described a series of 11 overweight men between the ages of 34 and 56 who possessed a constellation of findings including easily everted upper eyelids, papillary conjunctivitis, ocular irritation, and conjunctival keratinization. They noted that the ocular irritation correlated with sleeping preference in that men who predominantly slept on one side were affected in the ipsilateral eye. Men who slept face down often had bilateral involvement. Since the eyelids, conjunctiva, and cornea are affected in FES, it is a potentially blinding disorder. [2]

While FES has been more precisely described over the past three decades, the hallmark of the syndrome remains the easily everted upper eyelid. The chief presenting complaint of FES is chronic ocular irritation often accompanied by redness, foreign body sensation, dryness, photosensitivity, and mucous discharge. [3, 4] Unfortunately, these symptoms are not specific for FES and are consistent with more common conditions, such as dry eye syndrome and conjunctivitis As a result, proper diagnosis and treatment may be delayed. [3]

At rest, the eyelids of these patients usually contain redundant skin that may lead to eyelid ptosis, upper eyelid lash ptosis (Figure 2), and eyelash misalignment. [5, 6] Eyelids do not contain subcutaneous fat and must maintain rigidity in order to cover and protect the eye. This rigidity is mostly provided by the tarsal plate; however, in FES, the tarsal plates are easily foldable and the eyelid can be everted with minimal manual effort (Figures 1). [7] Evidence of chronic papillary conjunctivitis in the form of mucoid discharge may also be present. [5] Some authors have reported blepharochalasis and entropion. [2, 8]

Involvement of the cornea occurs in as many as 80 percent of patients with FES. [1, 9] Descriptions of corneal scarring with neovascularization have been widely reported. Prolonged eversion of the eyelid at night chronically irritates the conjunctiva and may eventually lead to exposure keratopathy. [5] Initially, superficial punctate keratopathy is a common finding in FES. [7] Keratoconus, filamentary keratitis, and infectious keratitis may be part of the constellation of findings in FES, but are not universally present. [7, 10, 11] The original description of FES [1] reiterated by Ezra and colleagues [5] includes many of the salient clinical features of the syndrome.

The most distinctive feature in each case was the rubbery, malleable upper tarsus. Any external upward force applied gently to the upper eyelid caused the tarsus to evert. none of the patients were aware of any previous ocular disease. In all cases large papillae covered the upper palpebral conjunctiva

To this description may be added the following: papillary conjunctivitis, easy eversion of the upper eyelid, discomfort, a rubbery and pliant tarsal plate. [5] Easy eversion of the upper eyelid is a subjective diagnostic criteria, but sufficient. [12] Nonetheless, eyelid laxity can be quantified by objective measurements such as anterior eyelid distraction and vertical lid pull tests. [2, 12, 13] Slit lamp examination of the affected eye may show hypertrophy of the superior palpebral tarsal conjunctiva, superior bulbar conjunctival injection, and paracentral thinning of the cornea consistent with keratoconus. [7, 10]

Demographic clues may help guide clinicians in making the diagnosis of FES. The syndrome still appears to be more common among overweight men in middle age (e.g., 40 – 69), similar to the original description. [5, 14] Nevertheless, the syndrome has been described in children, in women, and in people of normal weight. [7, 14-17] FES has been correlated with systemic conditions including obesity, hypertension, connective tissue disorders, glaucoma, ischemic heart disease, and anatomical/structural abnormalities of the cornea or eyelids. [4, 15] The strength of these correlations has been limited by relatively small sample sizes, however. In a series of 60 patients with FES, 18 percent had diabetes mellitus and 14 percent had hypertension. [7] In a series of 11 patients, the prevalence of hypertension and diabetes was 36.4 percent and nearly 20 percent had dyslipidemia. [18] All seven individuals suffering from Ehlers Danlos Syndrome (classic form, collagen V mutation) in one case series also had signs and symptoms consistent with FES. [15] In a separate study, 3 of 7 patients with FES had psoriasis, [19] a comorbidity that was also mentioned by other authors. [2, 18] Obstructive sleep apnea and FES commonly occur together. [2, 9, 20]

Floppy Eyelid Syndrome and Obstructive Sleep Apnea

The most commonly documented systemic illness related to FES is obstructive sleep apnea (OSA) Woog was the first to propose an association between the two conditions in 1990; [21] however, in 1987 Gonnering and Sonneland documented a patient with FES and symptoms consistent with OSA. [22] Since that time, several studies examining the association between FES and OSA have been published. [2, 12, 23-26] Retrospective reviews by McNab found OSA in 96 percent [25] and 100 percent[2] of patients with FES. Conversely, cross-sectional studies have yielded a low prevalence (4.5 percent [12] and 5 percent [2]) of FES in patients with OSA. Robert and colleagues reported increased eyelid laxity, though not necessarily FES, among individuals with OSA. [27]

In 2012, Chambe and coauthors reported on the results of a prospective case series including 127 individuals with suspected OSA syndrome. [24] Apnea severity was quantified with overnight polysomnography using an obstructive apnea-hypoxia index. As expected, body mass index, male gender, and age positively correlated with apnea severity. In this referred group, FES was identified in 15.8 percent of patients without demonstrable OSA and 25.8 percent of participants with OSA. When the group was stratified by apnea severity, 40 percent of individuals with severe apnea had FES. After correcting for known risk factors, there was a significant association between apnea severity and FES. [24]

In 2013, Muniesa prospectively followed 114 people admitted for OSA evaluation along with 45 patients with FES who were sent for polysomnography. [23] OSA was diagnosed in 89 patients, 14 (16 percent) of which also had FES. Interestingly, 54 (61 percent) had increased laxity of the upper eyelid. Twenty-five individuals did not have OSA, though FES was diagnosed in two of these individuals (8 percent) and eight had eyelid hyperlaxity (32 percent). The severity of OSA appears to be a critical factor in the development of FES. When authors restrict or stratify their cohort to include only individuals with severe OSA (e.g., apnea-hypoxia index greater than 30 per hour), the prevalence of FES ranges from 40 to 70 percent. [24, 26] Moreover, the prevalence of FES strongly correlates with measures of apnea severity, such as a respiratory distress index. [26]

The pathophysiology of FES is not clearly defined. In the original description of FES [1] and observed thereafter, [7] sleeping habits may predict which eye or eyes is affected. In other words, FES occurs predominantly in the eye that is "face down" during sleep Individuals without a strong sleeping preference, usually have symptoms and signs in both eyes. This has led many groups to postulate that chronic irritation during sleep at least contributes to the development and severity of FES. Likewise, eye shields and lid taping, which block this chronic irritation, are therapeutic in many individuals

Culbertson and Tseng proposed a causative relationship between apnea and FES. [7] They suggest compression of the eyelid, caused by sleeping face down on the affected eye, creates a relatively hypoxic environment in the eyelid. The hypoxia in the eyelid is further exacerbated by low oxygen tensions during sleep in individuals with sleep apnea Since people with sleep apnea often have fitful sleep and awaken frequently, the hypoxic eyelid has recurrent periods of reperfusion. This reperfusion after ischemia creates a cytotoxic microenvironment of oxygen free radical species that may damage the tarsus. [28] While this proposed mechanism has not yet been confirmed, it would be supported by the fact that treatment for sleep apnea (e.g., continuous positive airway pressure, CPAP) appears to be beneficial in FES. [29] Taken further, effective sleep apnea treatment may also be preventative in FES. [30] Conversely, the use of CPAP may alter sleeping position and consequent prevention of mechanical eversion of the eyelids. This, in turn, would improve initial symptoms

Given the laxity in the tarsal plate that occurs in FES, one may intuitively expect to find structural abnormalities. Initial histologic and ultrastructural studies by Dutton, [31] Goldberg, [8] and Arocker-Mettinger [32] in a small number of patients failed to show abnormalities in the connective tissue or in elastin or collagen fibers Histological studies with specialized staining techniques revealed that patients with FES may indeed have a loss of elastin in the tarsal plate. [33] Other components of the extracellular matrix such as glycosaminoglycans and proteoglycans were normal in this series. [33] Interestingly, this study highlighted a unique distribution of elastic fibers in the tarsal plate. Specifically, there is a relative paucity of elastin fibers in the stroma with normal or even increased numbers (and thickening) of elastin fibers around the meibomian acini. Several studies have failed to show significant abnormalities on collagen fiber numbers or density in FES, [18, 34] while confirming the decrease in elastin fibers. [18] Interestingly, skin samples taken from patients who have abnormal elastin fibers in their eyelids do not show the same pathology. [18] A newer study confirmed previous reports by showing decreased mature elastic fibers in the tarsal extracellular matrix, but also went a step further to show an increase in oxytalan fibers. [35] The authors postulated this to be an adaptive response to mechanical stress. [35] Slightly complicating the assumption that FES is a disorder of abnormal elastin is the finding that individuals with collagen V mutations (classic Ehlers Danlos Syndrome) seem to have a high incidence of FES. [15] This suggests a more primary role for collagen in the pathophysiology of the syndrome In summary, elastin and perhaps collagen abnormalities likely contribute to the pathophysiology of FES.

Relative deficiencies in elastin fibers in the tarsal plate and eyelid skin may be caused by increased lytic enzyme activity. Matrix metalloproteinases 7 and 9 are elastolytic and are upregulated in the syndrome. [18] These metalloproteinases are likely induced by repeated mechanical trauma and stress. [18] The intermittent hypoxia that occurs during apnea/hypopnea may trigger increased metalloproteinase activity, [36] though these links have yet to be shown empirically in FES. One particularly intriguing explanation for the increase in metalloproteinase 9 activity is hyperleptinemia. Patients with FES have elevated plasma leptin levels, positively correlating with body mass index. [37] Leptin stimulates metalloproteinase 9 in a dose-dependent manner. [38] Moreover, metalloproteinase 9 levels and activity are significantly higher in people with OSA. [39]

Leptin may serve as a mechanistic link between obesity, OSA, and FES. Further research in this arena will help to elucidate the underlying biochemical causes of this disease.

Several conservative treatments for FES have been proposed and implemented with varying degrees of success. In their original paper on the syndrome, Culbertson and Ostler taped the eyelids closed at night to prevent the upper eyelid from everting during sleep, which they found to be successful. [1] Nocturnal eye shields may also be helpful in some patients. [40] The use of topical agents such as lubricants, antibiotics, and steroids may be helpful in temporary symptomatic relief, infection, or severe inflammation; however, FES is notoriously resistant to topical treatments. [2, 9] Other medical treatments include lid scrubbing and punctual plugs. [5, 11]

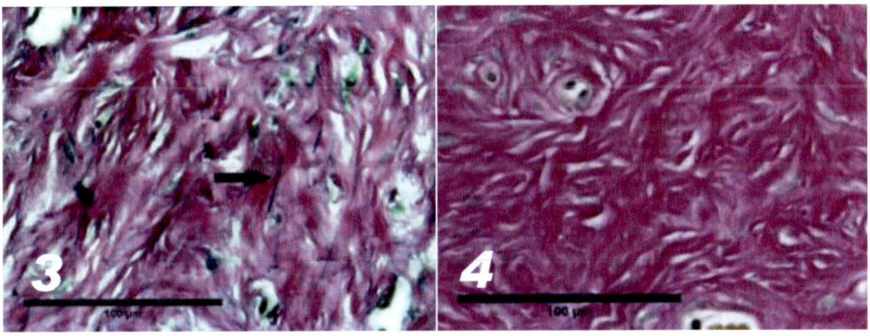

Intermeibomian matrix of tarsal plate tissue stained with Verhöeff's Iron Hematoxylin and Masson Trichrome counterstain. Figure 3. Note the presence of mature elastic fibers (black arrow) in normal tarsal plate. Figure 4. Note the absence of mature elastic fibers in tarsal plate tissue of patient with floppy eyelid syndrome (Photo credit: Ezra, D. G., Ellis, J. S., et al. (2011), Changes in tarsal plate fibrillar collagens and elastic fibre phenotype in floppy eyelid syndrome. Clinical and Experimental Ophthalmology, 39: 564–571.)

While conservative medical treatments are considered first-line therapy for FES, many patients are unable to consistently adhere to nocturnal taping or eye shields. Consequently, patients and clinicians often turn to surgical correction of the eyelid. Full-thickness wedge excision has been described in over a dozen papers (for review see Ezra et al. [5]). In this procedure, also known as pentagon excision, incisions are made perpendicular to the lid margin and a full thickness section of the eyelid is removed. Several authors have reported 100 percent success rates at follow-up of up to three years. [2, 41] The standard full-thickness wedge excision may be enhanced for cosmetic effect by back tapering the incision to disguise the scar. [41] In this approach, the lateral canthal tendon is not disrupted. The lateral tarsal strip procedure was developed as a treatment for lower lid laxity though it is been adapted for use in FES. [17, 42] Data on the short and long-term success of the lateral tarsal strip in FES is limited. Success rates above 90 percent have been reported in the treatment of lax eyelid syndrome. [43]

Various other surgical techniques have been described including lateral tarsorrhaphy, lateral canthal tendon plication, and modified Bick's procedure. Bouchard was the first to publish on lateral tarsorrhaphy for patients who could not comply with eye shielding. [44] In lateral tarsorrhaphy, the lateral portions of the eyelids are partially sutured together to reduce the palpebral aperture. In lateral canthal tendon plication, lateral end of the tarsal plate is sutured to the periosteum of the lateral orbital wall, which spares the tendon without reconstruction. [45] Despite widespread use of lateral canthal tendon plication, very few long-term data on the success of this approach are available. The modified Bick's procedure combines a classic Bick (full thickness trapezoid incision at the lateral canthus) with a lateral tarsal strip procedure. [46] Short-term success rates are extremely high (90 percent or higher), but long-term results are conspicuously absent from the literature.

Periman's lateral full-thickness wedge excision with back tapering appears to provide excellent long-term success with a relatively cosmetically favorable result. [41] On the other hand, Ezra and colleagues reviewed the results of 71 FES patients treated with various surgical interventions over 13 years. [47] Their major endpoint was recurrence of the condition as evidenced by two independent observers who are unaware of the surgical assignment of the study participants. In this series, superior survival outcomes (e.g., durable surgical result without a return of FES symptoms) were achieved with medial and lateral canthal tendon plication and upper eyelid lateral tarsal strip compared to full-thickness wedge excision. [47] There was no significant difference between canthal plication and lateral tarsal strip procedures nor were there significant differences in outcomes between surgeons or surgical teams Full-thickness wedge excision failed to deliver a durable result in 60.6 percent of patients treated with this surgical approach. On the other hand, failure rates for medial/lateral canthal plication were 47 percent and 25.6 percent, respectively. The researchers also found that patients who did not have a recurrence of FES in the first 2 to 4 years after surgery would almost certainly remain symptom free. [47] Ezra and co-authors recommend using lateral tarsal strip for patients that either have a relatively isolated lateral canthal laxity or no canthal laxity. This seemingly disparate set of recommendations follows from the fact that lateral tarsal strip tightens the tarsal plate with minimal sacrifice of tarsal tissue Furthermore, they recommend medial/lateral canthal plication for people with both medial and lateral canthal laxity. A medial canthal strip procedure (33.3 percent failure rate) is recommended for patients with predominantly medial canthal laxity. [47]

For individuals with FES, it is reasonable to consider polysomnography or a "sleep study" to investigate possible presence of OSA. [30] Indeed, it is possible that OSA is an independent risk factor for FES. [23] More importantly, treating OSA may also improve FES. For example, McNab reported the case of an obese 32-year-old man with both conditions who failed treatment with eye shields. The man enjoyed a full resolution of his FES symptoms after treatment with a CPAP device. [29] Lid laxity completely disappeared and he no longer had evidence of conjunctival irritation. [29] The beneficial effect of CPAP has been reported in larger cohorts as well. [25] In fact, patients with both FES and OSA who had surgical correction of the eyelid without definitive treatment for apnea tended to have a recurrence of eye symptoms.

The overall success rate of medical and surgical treatment of FES varies substantially. Most studies suffer from inadequate long-term follow-up periods and small cohort sizes. Nevertheless, most patients can expect to benefit from either medical or surgical treatment. [9] OSA should be aggressively treated because it is a potentially fatal condition but also may improve symptoms of FES. FES may be a presenting complaint of people with undiagnosed sleep apnea It is also reasonable to assume that weight loss may be helpful for both conditions.

Acknowledgment

Ginger Roberts, MLS, Research and Liaison Librarian for assistance with image acquisition.

References

[1] Culbertson W. W, Ostler H. B. The floppy eyelid syndrome *Am. J. Ophthalmol.,* 1981; 92:568-75.
[2] McNab A. A. Floppy eyelid syndrome and obstructive sleep apnea *Ophthal. Plast. Reconstr. Surg.,* 1997; 13:98-114.
[3] Pham T. T., Perry J. D. Floppy eyelid syndrome *Curr. Opin. Ophthalmol.,* 2007; 18:430-3.
[4] Miyamoto C., Espirito Santo L. C., Roisman L., Moreno Pde A., Cariello A. J., Osaki M. H. Floppy eyelid syndrome: review. *Arq. Bras. Oftalmol.,* 2011; 74:64-6.
[5] Ezra D. G., Beaconsfield M., Collin R. Floppy eyelid syndrome: stretching the limits. *Surv. Ophthalmol.,* 2010; 55:35-46.
[6] Langford J. D., Linberg J. V. A new physical finding in floppy eyelid syndrome *Ophthalmology,* 1998; 105:165-9.
[7] Culbertson W. W., Tseng S. C. Corneal disorders in floppy eyelid syndrome *Cornea,* 1994; 13:33-42.
[8] Goldberg R., Seiff S., McFarland J., Simons K., Shorr N. Floppy eyelid syndrome and blepharochalasis. *Am. J. Ophthalmol.,* 1986; 102:376-81.

[9] Leibovitch I., Selva D. Floppy eyelid syndrome: clinical features and the association with obstructive sleep apnea *Sleep Med.,* 2006; 7:117-22.

[10] Donnenfeld E. D., Perry H. D., Gibralter R. P., Ingraham H. J., Udell I. J. Keratoconus associated with floppy eyelid syndrome *Ophthalmology,* 1991; 98:1674-8.

[11] Diller R., Sant S. A case report and review of filamentary keratitis. *Optometry,* 2005; 76:30-6.

[12] Karger R. A., White W. A., Park W. C., et al. Prevalence of floppy eyelid syndrome in obstructive sleep apnea-hypopnea syndrome. *Ophthalmology,* 2006; 113:1669-74.

[13] Iyengar S. S., Khan J. A. Quantifying upper eyelid laxity in symptomatic floppy eyelid syndrome by measurement of anterior eyelid distraction. *Ophthal. Plast. Reconstr. Surg.,* 2007; 23:255.

[14] Brown M. D., Potter J. W. Floppy eyelid syndrome: a case report and clinical review. *J. Am. Optom. Assoc.,* 1992; 63:309-14.

[15] Segev F., Heon E., Cole W. G., et al. Structural abnormalities of the cornea and lid resulting from collagen V mutations *Invest. Ophthalmol. Vis. Sci.,* 2006; 47:565-73.

[16] Gerner E. W., Hughes S. M. Floppy eyelid with hyperglycinemia. *Am. J. Ophthalmol.,* 1984; 98:614-6.

[17] Eiferman R. A., Gossman M. D., O'Neill K., Douglas C. H. Floppy eyelid syndrome in a child. *Am. J. Ophthalmol.,* 1990; 109:356-7.

[18] Schlotzer-Schrehardt U., Stojkovic M., Hofmann-Rummelt C., Cursiefen C., Kruse F. E., Holbach L. M. The Pathogenesis of floppy eyelid syndrome: involvement of matrix metalloproteinases in elastic fiber degradation *Ophthalmology,* 2005; 112:694-704.

[19] Schwartz L. K., Gelender H., Forster R. K. Chronic conjunctivitis associated with 'floppy eyelids'. *Arch. Ophthalmol.,* 1983; 101:1884-8.

[20] Karhanova M., Hobzova M., Maresova K. [Floppy eyelid syndrome and obstructive sleep apnoea]. *Cesk. Slov. Oftalmol.,* 2012; 68:22-6, 28.

[21] Woog J. J. Obstructive sleep apnea and the floppy eyelid syndrome *Am. J. Ophthalmol.,* 1990; 110:314-5.

[22] Gonnering R. S., Sonneland P. R. Meibomian gland dysfunction in floppy eyelid syndrome *Ophthal. Plast. Reconstr. Surg.,* 1987; 3:99-103.

[23] Muniesa M. J., Huerva V., Sanchez-de-la-Torre M., Martinez M., Jurjo C., Barbe F. The relationship between floppy eyelid syndrome and obstructive sleep apnoea. *Br. J. Ophthalmol.,* 2013; 97:1387-90.

[24] Chambe J., Laib S., Hubbard J., et al. Floppy eyelid syndrome is associated with obstructive sleep apnoea: a prospective study on 127 patients. *J. Sleep Res.*, 2012; 21:308-15.

[25] McNab A. A. The eye and sleep *Clin. Experiment. Ophthalmol.*, 2005; 33:117-25.

[26] Mojon D. S., Goldblum D., Fleischhauer J., et al. Eyelid, conjunctival, and corneal findings in sleep apnea syndrome *Ophthalmology*, 1999;106:1182-5.

[27] Robert P. Y., Adenis J. P., Tapie P., Melloni B. Eyelid hyperlaxity and obstructive sleep apnea (O.S.A.) syndrome *Eur. J. Ophthalmol.*, 1997; 7:211-5.

[28] Sussman M. S., Bulkley G. B. Oxygen-derived free radicals in reperfusion injury *Methods Enzymol.*, 1990; 186:711-23.

[29] McNab A. A. Reversal of floppy eyelid syndrome with treatment of obstructive sleep apnoea. *Clin. Experiment. Ophthalmol.*, 2000; 28: 125-6.

[30] McNab A. A. The eye and sleep apnea *Sleep Med. Rev.*, 2007; 11: 269-76.

[31] Dutton J. J. Surgical management of floppy eyelid syndrome *Am. J. Ophthalmol.*, 1985; 99:557-60.

[32] Arocker-Mettinger E., Haddad R., Konrad K., Steinkogler F. J. [Floppy eyelid syndrome: light and electron microscopy studies]. *Klin. Monbl. Augenheilkd.*, 1986; 188:596-8.

[33] Netland P. A., Sugrue S. P., Albert D. M., Shore J. W. Histopathologic features of the floppy eyelid syndrome Involvement of tarsal elastin *Ophthalmology*, 1994; 101:174-81.

[34] Valenzuela A. A., Sullivan T. J. Medial upper eyelid shortening to correct medial eyelid laxity in floppy eyelid syndrome: a new surgical approach. *Ophthal. Plast. Reconstr. Surg.*, 2005; 21:259-63.

[35] Ezra D. G., Ellis J. S., Gaughan C., et al. Changes in tarsal plate fibrillar collagens and elastic fibre phenotype in floppy eyelid syndrome *Clinical and Experimental Ophthalmology*, 2011; 39(6):564–571.

[36] Kondo S., Kubota S., Shimo T., et al. Connective tissue growth factor increased by hypoxia may initiate angiogenesis in collaboration with matrix metalloproteinase s. *Carcinogenesis*, 2002; 23:769-76.

[37] Taban M., Taban M., Perry J. D. Plasma leptin levels in patients with floppy eyelid syndrome *Ophthalmic Plastic and Reconstructive Surgery*, 2006; 22:375-377.

[38] Castellucci M., De Matteis R., Meisser A., et al. Leptin modulates extracellular matrix molecules and metalloproteinases: possible implications for trophoblast invasion. *Mol. Hum. Reprod.,* 2000; 6: 951-8.

[39] Tazaki T., Minoguchi K., Yokoe T., et al. Increased levels and activity of matrix metalloproteinase-9 in obstructive sleep apnea syndrome *American journal of respiratory and critical care medicine,* 2004; 170: 1354-1359.

[40] Parunovic A. Floppy eyelid syndrome *Br. J. Ophthalmol.,* 1983; 67: 264-6.

[41] Periman L. M., Sires B. S. Floppy eyelid syndrome: a modified surgical technique *Ophthal. Plast. Reconstr. Surg.,* 2002; 18:370-2.

[42] Viana G. A., Sant'Anna A. E., Righetti F., Osaki M. Floppy eyelid syndrome *Plast. Reconstr. Surg.,* 2008; 121:333e-334e.

[43] Burkat C. N., Lemke B. N. Acquired lax eyelid syndrome: an unrecognized cause of the chronically irritated eye. *Ophthal. Plast. Reconstr. Surg.,* 2005; 21:52-8.

[44] Bouchard C. S. Lateral tarsorrhaphy for a noncompliant patient with floppy eyelid syndrome *Am. J. Ophthalmol.,* 1992; 114:367-9.

[45] Karesh J. W., Nirankari V. S., Hameroff S. B. Eyelid imbrication. An unrecognized cause of chronic ocular irritation. *Ophthalmology,* 1993; 100:883-9.

[46] Barrett R. V., Meyer D. R. The modified Bick quick strip procedure for surgical treatment of eyelid malposition. *Ophthal. Plast. Reconstr. Surg.,* 2012; 28:294-9.

[47] Ezra D. G., Beaconsfield M., Sira M., et al. Long-term outcomes of surgical approaches to the treatment of floppy eyelid syndrome *Ophthalmology,* 2010; 117:839-46.

In: Eye Diseases …
Editor: Mingwu Wang
ISBN: 978-1-63482-894-9

Chapter 3

Dry Eye Disease and Sleep Deprivation

Joshua K. Duncan, DO and Mingwu Wang*, MD, PhD
Department of Ophthalmology and Vision Science,
University of Arizona College of Medicine, AZ, US

Case Presentation

A young male graduate student presents for evaluation of intermittent blurry vision, ocular irritation, foreign body sensation, and redness. He reports having been sleeping only a few hours each night for the past several weeks to prepare for his final exams. His symptoms appeared and have been worsening during this time. Slit-lamp biomicroscopy reveals diffuse conjunctival injection (Figure 1), punctate fluorescein staining of the cornea (Figure 2), and a short tear break up time in both eyes. Tear osmolarity is measured to be 332 mOsmol/L in the right eye and 328 mOsmol/L in the left eye. The Schirmer test is 9 mm in each eye. He is diagnosed with dry eyes and prescribed artificial tears for lubrication. The importance of adequate sleep to allow good rest of the eyes daily is also discussed with the patient.

* E-mail: mwang@eyes.arizona.edu.

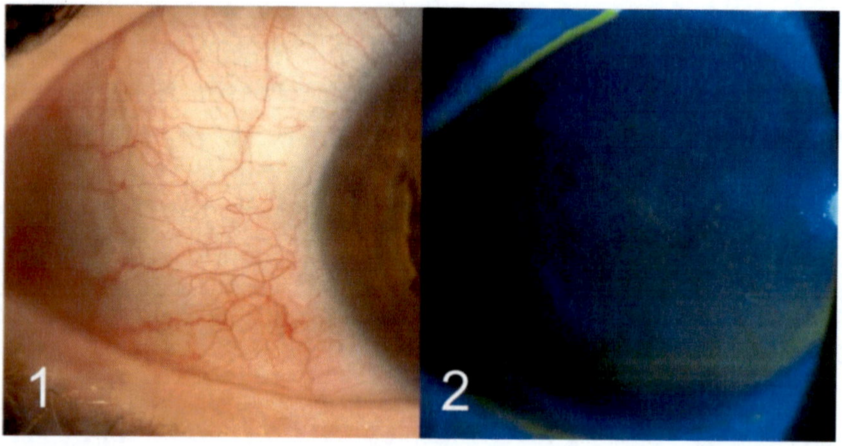

Figure 1. Dilation of fine subconjunctival vessels in a patient with chronic sleep deprivation. Figure 2. Corneal fluorescein staining showing diffuse punctate epithelial erosions characteristically seen in dry eye syndrome.

Dry Eye Syndrome: An Overview

Dry eye syndrome (DES), also known as keratoconjunctivitis sicca, is a common condition that accounts for a significant percentage of ophthalmologic visits each year. As the population ages, its prevalence is expected to increase as is the burden on ophthalmologic practices. [1] In fact, currently in the United States, up to 10-30 percent of the population older than 40 may be afflicted with this condition. [2] It is estimated that 3.23 million women and 1.68 million men over the age of 50 have signs and symptoms of dry eyes, and undoubtedly many more are undiagnosed. [2]

DES is a multifactorial disease of the tears and the ocular surface that results in discomfort, visual disturbance, tear film instability, and inflammation. [3] Symptoms of dry eye most commonly include burning, itching, irritation, foreign body sensation, redness, tearing, blurred vision, photosensitivity, and discharge. [4] Symptoms can be unilateral or bilateral, and tend to be worse toward the end of the day, with prolonged use of the eyes, or with exposure to extreme environmental conditions. Several factors including computer use, air conditioning, contact lenses, refractive surgery, as well as medications (e.g., antihistamines and hormonal therapy) have been implicated in the development and severity of dry eyes. [1, 5] DES can occur as an isolated finding, but is often associated with systemic rheumatologic, infectious, and inflammatory disease. [6] Health care providers should be cognizant of dry eye complaints, their association with systemic diseases, and refer patients for further testing and treatment Left untreated, this condition has the potential to cause long-term damage and permanent vision loss.

DES is currently classified into two general categories, aqueous deficient or evaporative dry eyes. [3] Aqueous deficiency is thought to be caused by insufficient tears secreted by the main and accessory lacrimal glands, which are regulated by the parasympathetic nervous system. [7] In the evaporative form, intrinsic and extrinsic factors lead to excessive loss of tears from the ocular surface, and subsequent dryness develops. Intrinsic factors include meibomian gland dysfunction (MGD), decreased blink rate, and disorders of the eyelid, including floppy eyelid syndrome (FES). Extrinsic causes of evaporative dry eye include preexisting ocular surface disease, allergies, and contact lens wear. [8]

A thorough ophthalmologic evaluation is warranted when patients present with symptoms of dry eyes The most common objective measures used to evaluate corneal surface abnormalities are tear break up time (TBUT), corneal staining, tear osmolarity, and the Schirmer test. [9] The tear film must be redistributed with each blink. Normally, this happens approximately 17 times per minute at rest. [10] The TBUT is measured using a cobalt blue light source to view the tear film after instillation of fluorescein dye. The first appearance of a dark spot in the tear film signifies the beginning of tear break-up. A TBUT of less than 10 seconds represents instability, and is indicative of dry eye. [3] Corneal staining is used to identify surface irregularities or signs of devitalized epithelium Various stain patterns can be a clue to the investigators as to the etiology of the underlying disorder The degree of cornea staining usually correlates with the severity of the dry eye. [3] Tear osmolarity also plays a significant role in the pathogenesis of dry eyes. Tear hyperosmolarity may occur as a result of increased evaporation or reduced aqueous secretion

Several devices are available for use in the clinical setting that can determine osmolarity of tears by using electrical impedance; values above 312 mOsmol/L indicate moderate to severe dry eyes. [8] The Schirmer test, also frequently used in the evaluation of dry eyes, involves application of a filter paper wick into the lower conjunctival sac and measurement of the wetting length over 5 minutes. Values less than 10 mm usually signify the presence of dry eyes.

The pathogenesis of DES is multifactorial. Two hallmarks involved in the disease process are tear hyperosmolarity and inflammation As the osmolarity of the tear film increases, inflammatory changes occur, resulting in damage to the epithelium of the ocular surface. [11-13] An increase in tear osmolarity is common to all types of dry eyes, regardless of the etiology The degree of inflammation seen on the ocular surface also appears to be related to the severity of DES. One study showed that elevated levels of inflammatory cytokines such as IL-1, IL-6, IL-8, TNF -α and TGF -β in the tears from patients with dry eyes correlated with the severity of the disease. [14] Effective treatment of dry eyes is dictated by addressing both the inflammation and the abnormal tear osmolarity. Further studies are needed to clarify the exact role these inflammatory mediators play in the pathogenesis of the disease, and could potentially provide specific targets for therapeutic intervention in the future.

Sleep Deprivation, Dry Eyes and Ocular Surface Disease

Sleep plays a vital role in our overall health Insufficient sleep, or poor quality of sleep has been linked to increased incidence of cardiovascular disease, obesity, diabetes, impaired immune function, as well as changes on the ocular surface. [15, 16-19] It is well recognized clinically that lack of sleep leads to red eyes, but sleep deprivation may have an even more significant impact on the ocular surface than we had originally thought. One recent study looked at sleep deprivation and its effects on the ocular surface in healthy young subjects with no prior evidence of dry eyes In this study, 10 subjects were prohibited from sleeping for 24 hours, while 10 control subjects were allowed to sleep for 8 hours. A thorough ophthalmic examination, conducted on both groups, showed that sleep deprivation caused increased tear osmolarity, decreased TBUT, and decreased tear secretion by the Schirmer test. [15] Patients subjected to sleep deprivation also reported significantly more symptoms including discomfort, dryness, and foreign body sensation. [15] Further evidence that inadequate sleep leads to dry eyes is seen in another study that looked at healthy high school students. [20] Subjects were interviewed to determine sleep habits and presence of ocular symptoms. Ophthalmic examinations were then conducted to screen for dry eyes. They found that students with poor sleep quality were 1.342 times more likely than those without to have dry eyes. [20]

It is now thought that sleep deprivation or poor sleep quality may directly cause or exacerbate dry eyes in susceptible patients. Several mechanisms have been postulated to explain these findings. First, the parasympathetic nervous system controls tear production in the lacrimal gland. [3, 15, 21] Sleep deprivation is believed to lead to higher levels of stress hormones, including cortisol, epinephrine, and norepinephrine, and to decrease parasympathetic and increase sympathetic tones. [22-24] This relative decrease of parasympathetic tone presumably causes less tear production and exacerbates dry eyes. Additionally, the properties of the tear film undergo a change during extended periods of eye closure The human tear film has a lower osmolarity and increased immunoglobulins upon waking compared to that present immediately before sleep. [25-27] Lack of sleep, or insufficient sleep would inevitably affect the quality of tears and worsen dry eye symptoms. [25] Moreover, tear secretion may be influenced by hormonal factors in sleep derivation. Lack of sleep leads to mild activation of the hypothalamic–pituitary–adrenal axis with subsequent elevation of plasma glucocorticoids and mineralocorticoids. [28-30] This causes diuresis and natriuresis through the renin –angiotensin–aldosterone system which could cause a relative dehydration and reduced tear secretion. [30] In addition, prolonged opening of eyes would promote the evaporation of tears form the ocular surface and exacerbate dry eyes. It is plausible to believe that eye closure during sleep provides an opportunity for the restoration of the homeostatic tears at the ocular surface. Any interruption of this process would cause abnormalities of the tear film and adverse consequences to the ocular surface.

Conditions such as obstructive sleep apnea (OSA), which is characterized by recurrent sympathetic nervous system activation and arousal from sleep, essentially lead to chronic sleep deprivation. [31] Patients with OSA are particularly prone to DES and other ocular surface disorders. Frequently, it is the ocular complications that lead to discomfort and visual impairment, which prompts patients to seek medical evaluation.

There are several external eye and corneal findings associated with OSA. These include FES, lid ptosis, ectropion, punctate epithelial keratopathy, papillary conjunctivitis, recurrent corneal erosions, keratoconus, and DES. [32, 33] Although many of these lid and ocular surface findings are hypothesized to be secondary to the FES and the mechanical effects of eyelid malposition during sleep, there is increasing evidence that points to lack of sleep as a primary cause for the ocular surface disease. [15, 34, 35]

The association of FES with OSA has been well established with an estimated prevalence as high as 31 percent in several studies. [34, 36] Despite this, as a condition of lax and easily everted eyelids with a pliable, soft tarsus, FES is likely still under-diagnosed. [4] OSA and FES play a critical role in the pathogenesis of corneal surface disease and dry eyes Poor lid apposition and abnormal lid-tear interface leads to corneal and conjunctival breakdown in as high as 71 percent of patients. [33] The nocturnal exposure of the ocular surface places them at an increased risk for infection, inflammatory response, and frequently, significant dry eye symptoms.

Patients with OSA will often present for medical care with symptoms of dry eyes Symptoms are generally worse on the side on which patients prefer to sleep This is supported by the presence of asymmetrical disease corresponding to sleep posture, and the resolution of symptoms with the use of an eye shield. [35, 37] Dry eye subjects and those with FES caused by OSA have been shown to exhibit tear film instability, and decreased TBUT. [32, 38] One study has shown correlation between an advanced-type corneal staining pattern and the severity of OSA. [39] Moreover, the Schirmer test has been conducted in patients with OSA and FES, and lower values have been associated with more advanced disease. [39]

In patients with OSA, it is the mechanical effects relating upper lid laxity, exposure of the corneal and conjunctival surface, that are thought to play the most significant role in the evaporative loss of tears. However, other mechanisms such as MGD, upregulation of elastolytic enzymes, and local ischemia, have also been proposed to account for the ocular surface disease seen in these patients. [33, 40-42]

Meibomian glands are sebaceous glands located in the tarsal plate of the upper and lower eyelids. They are found on the mucocutaneous lid junction, emptying their lipid contents (meibum) onto the ocular surface in a holocrine fashion. This meibum functions to prevent evaporation of the aqueous layer of the tear film. MGD is often found commonly in patients with OSA, and its symptoms often mimic that of DES. *Gonnering and Sooneland* showed this by examining a histologic sample of the tarsal plate from a patient who underwent upper eyelid surgery for the treatment of FES. [40] They found keratinization extending well up the meibomian ducts, with squamous metaplasia and granuloma formation within the acini. These findings were identical to that seen in MGD, and were hypothesized to be secondary to floppy eyelids. [40]

The mechanical injury to the ocular surface, seen in patients with OSA and FES, is not simply caused by eye rubbing and noctural lid eversion. In fact, histopathologic studies of eyelid biopsy specimens have described decreased amounts of elastin fibers in the tarsal plate of patients with floppy eyelids. [43] A study showed that this was due to increased expression of elastin-degrading enzymes, particularly matrix metalloproteinase (MMP)-7 and -9, in the tarsus and the eyelids. [41] It was postulated that these lytic enzymes were up-regulated in patients with OSA secondary to chronic mechanical irritation, local inflammation, and ischemia with subsequent reperfusion injury. [41] Proper contact of the eyelids with the cornea during sleep is essential for nourishment of the cornea, and the maintenance of a healthy tear film.

In summary, it is likely a constellation of factors including poor sleep quality, nocturnal eversion and poor contact of the eyelids with the ocular surface from elastic fiber degradation and tissue damage, in conjunction with meibomian gland and tear film abnormalities that lead to significant ocular morbidity in these patients.

Treatment of dry eyes frequently involves several modalities and a multidisciplinary approach. The cornerstones of treatment involve keeping the ocular surface moist, and controlling local and systemic inflammation Tear substitutes, gels and ointments are used for lubrication and to allow time for epithelial repair Steroid eye drops can be used short-term as a bridging therapy for severe ocular surface inflammation. Oral tetracycline therapy has been shown to inhibit elastolytic enzymes (e.g., MMPs), and therefore indicated in the treatment of coexisting MGD. Nighttime patching, taping, eye masks, shields, or the use of removable lid weights can limit evaporative tear loss during sleep. [4] Topical cyclosporine A, an immunomodulatory agent, has been shown to increase tear production and be effective for moderate to severe dry eyes. [44, 45]

In addition to local measures, chronic sleep deprivation should be considered as an etiology for patients with recalcitrant DES. Proper assessment of sleep disorders is imperative for the decision on a proper treatment Effective treatment of OSA, most commonly using continuous positive airway pressure (CPAP) devices, as well as weight loss have been shown to alleviate ocular symptoms caused by FES. [46] In fact, in several studies, proper CPAP use lead to regression of floppy eyelids, less ocular irritation, and improved tear film and overall corneal health. [34, 39] Conversely, poorly fit masks can lead to air leaks which have been implicated in several studies to cause worsening of corneal surface disease, conjunctival metaplasia, and even severe infections on occasion. [47, 48] For this reason, it is important for healthcare professionals to educate patients on the possible complications related to CPAP use, including the increased risks of ocular infection and the increased need for nocturnal lubrication to prevent dryness.

References

[1] Yagci A., Gurdal C. The role and treatment of inflammation in dry eye disease. *Int. Ophthalmol.*, 2014; 34:1291-301.

[2] The epidemiology of dry eye disease: Report of the Epidemiology Subcommittee of the International Dry Eye WorkShop (2007). *Ocul. Surf.*, 2007; 5:93-107.

[3] Lemp M. A. The definition and classification of dry eye disease: Report of the Definition and Classification Subcommittee of the International Dry Eye WorkShop. *Ocul. Surf.*, 2007; 5:75-92.

[4] Mastrota K. M. Impact of floppy eyelid syndrome in ocular surface and dry eye disease. *Optom. Vis. Sci.*, 2008; 85:814-16.

[5] Miljanovic B., Dana R., Sullivan D. A., Schaumberg D. A. Impact of dry eye syndrome on vision-related quality of life *Am. J. Ophthalmol.*, 2007; 143:409–15.

[6] Pflugfelder S. C. Antiinflammatory therapy for dry eye. *Am. J. Ophthalmol.*, 2004; 137:337-42.

[7] McGinnigle S., Naroo S. A., Eperjesi F. Evaluation of dry eye. *Surv. Ophthalmol.*, 2012; 57:293–316.

[8] Lemp M. A., Bron A. J., Baudouin C., et al. Tear osmolarity in the diagnosis and management of dry eye disease. *Am. J. Ophthalmol.*, 2011; 151:792-8.

[9] Serin D., Karsloglu S., Kyan A., et al. A simple approach to the repeatability of the schirmer test without anesthesia: eyes open or closed? *Cornea,* 2007; 26:903-6.

[10] Bentivoglio A. R., Bressman S. B., Cassetta E., et al. Analysis of blink rate patterns in normal subjects. *Mov. Disord.*, 1997; 12:1028-34.

[11] Bron A., Tiffany J., Yokoi N., et al. Using osmolarity to diagnose dry eye: a compartmental hypothesis and review of our assumptions. *Adv. Exp. Med. Biol.,* 2002; 506:1087-95.

[12] Farris R. L. Tear osmolarity – a new gold standard. *Adv. Exp. Med. Biol.*, 1994; 350:495-503.

[13] Tomlinson A., Khanal S., Ramaesh K., et al. Tear film osmolarity: determination of a referent for dry eye diagnosis. *Invest. Ophthalmol. Vis. Sci.,* 2006; 47:4309-15.

[14] Pflugfelder S. C., Jones D., Ji Z., et al. Altered cytokine balance in the tear fluid and conjunctiva of patients with Sjogren's syndrome keratoconjunctivitis sicca *Curr. Eye Res.*, 1999; 19:201-11.

[15] Lee Y. B., Koh J. W., Hyon J. Y., et al. Sleep deprivation reduces tear secretion and impairs the tear film. *Invest. Ophthalmol. Vis. Sci.,* 2014; 55:3525–31.

[16] Kohatsu N. D., et al. Sleep Duration and Body Mass Index in a Rural Population. *Archives of Internal Medicine*, 2006; 166: 1701-5.

[17] Knutson K. L., et al. Role of Sleep Duration and Quality in the Risk and Severity of Type 2 Diabetes Mellitus. *Archives of Internal Medicine,* 2006; 166:1768-74.

[18] King, C. R. et al. Short Sleep Duration and Incident Coronary Artery Calcification. *JAMA,* 2008; 300: 2859-66.

[19] Opp, M. R., et al. Neural-Immune Interactions in the Regulation of Sleep. *Front. Biosci.*, 2003; 8:768-79.

[20] Zhang Y., Chen H., Wu X. Prevalence and risk factors associated with dry eye syndrome among senior high school students in a county of Shandong Province, China *Ophthalmic Epidemiol.*, 2012; 19:226-30.

[21] Spiegel K., Leproult R., Van Cauter E. Impact of sleep debt on metabolic and endocrine function. *Lancet*, 1999; 354:1435–39.

[22] Nascimento D. C., Andersen M. L., Hip´olide D. C., et al. Pain hypersensitivity induced by paradoxical sleep deprivation is not due to altered binding to brain mu-opioid receptors *Behav. Brain Res.,* 2007; 178:216–20.

[23] Von Treuer K., Norman T. R., Armstrong S. M. Overnight human plasma melatonin, cortisol, prolactin, TSH, under conditions of normal sleep, sleep deprivation, and sleep recovery *J. Pineal Res.*, 1996; 20: 7–14.

[24] Dartt D. A. Regulation of tear secretion *Adv. Exp. Med. Biol.,* 1994; 350:1–9.

[25] Bitton E., Keech A., Jones L., et al. Subjective and objective variation of the tear film pre- and post-sleep *Optom. Vis. Sci.,* 2008 Aug.; 85:740-9.

[26] Terry J. E., Hill R. M. Human tear osmotic pressure: diurnal variations and the closed eye. *Arch. Ophthalmol.*, 1978; 96:120–2.

[27] Sack R. A., Tan K. O., Tan A. Diurnal tear cycle: evidence for a nocturnal inflammatory constitutive tear fluid *Invest. Ophthalmol. Vis. Sci.*, 1992; 33:626–40.

[28] Dartt D. A. Neural regulation of lacrimal gland secretory processes: relevance in dry eye diseases *Prog. Retin. Eye Res.,* 2009; 28:155–77.

[29] Dartt D. A. Regulation of tear secretion *Adv. Exp. Med. Biol.,* 1994; 350:1 9.

[30] Mahler B., Kamperis K., Schroeder M., et al. Sleep deprivation induces excess diuresis and natriuresis in healthy children *Am. J. Physiol. Renal Physiol.*, 2012; 302:236–43.

[31] Guilleminault C., Van den Hoed J., Mitler M. Clinical overview of the sleep apnea syndromes. In: Guilleminault C., Dement W. C., eds. Sleep Apnea Syndromes. New York: A.R. Liss, 1978;1–12.

[32] Mojon D. S., Goldblum D., Fleischhauer J., et al. Eyelid, conjunctival, and corneal findings in sleep apnea syndrome *Ophthalmology,* 1999; 106:1182–5.

[33] Culbertson W. W., Tseng S. C. Corneal disorders in floppy eyelid syndrome *Cornea,* 1994; 13:33–42.

[34] Kadyan A., Asghar J., Dowson L., et al. Ocular findings in sleep apnoea patients using continuous positive airway pressure *Eye (Lond.),* 2010; 24: 843–50.

[35] Donnenfeld E. D., Perry H. D., Gibralter R. P., et al. Keratoconus associated with floppy eyelid syndrome *Ophthalmology*, 1991;98: 1674–8.

[36] Chambe J., Laib S., Hubbard J., et al. Floppy eyelid syndrome is associated with obstructive sleep apnoea: a prospective study on 127 patients. *J. Sleep Res.,* 2012; 21:308–31.

[37] McNab A. A. Floppy eyelid syndrome and obstructive sleep apnea *Ophthal. Plast. Reconstr. Surg.*, 1997; 13:98–114.

[38] Liu D. T., Di Pascuale M. A., Sawai J., et al. Tear film dynamics in floppy eyelid syndrome *Invest. Ophthalmol. Vis. Sci.,* 2005; 46: 1188–94.

[39] Acar M., Firat H., Acar U., et al. Ocular surface assessment in patients with obstructive sleep apnea-hypopnea syndrome *Sleep Breath,* 2013; 17:583-8.

[40] Gonnering R. S., Sonneland P. R. Meibomian gland dysfunction in floppy eyelid syndrome *Ophthal. Plast. Reconstr. Surg.*, 1987;3:99–103.

[41] Schlotzer-Schrehardt U., Stojkovic M., Hofmann-Rummelt C., et al. The pathogenesis of floppy eyelid syndrome: involvement of matrix metalloproteinases in elastic fiber degradation *Ophthalmology,* 2005; 112:694–704.

[42] Van Nouhuys H. M., Van den Bosch W. A., Lemij H. G., et al. Floppy eyelid syndrome associated with demodex brevis *Orbit,* 1994; 13: 125–9.

[43] Netland P. A., Sugrue S. P., Albert D. M., et al. Histopathologic features of the floppy eyelid syndrome *Involvement of tarsal elastin Ophthalmology,* 1994; 101:174-81.

[44] Power W. J., Mullaney P., Farrell M., et al. Effect of topical cyclosporin A on conjunctival T cells in patients with secondary Sjögren's syndrome *Cornea,* 1993; 12:507–11.

[45] Sall K., Stevenson O. D., Mundorf T. K., et al. Two multicenter, randomized studies of the efficacy and safety of cyclosporine ophthalmic emulsion in moderate to severe dry eye disease. CsA Phase 3 Study Group. *Ophthalmology*, 2000; 107:631-9.

[46] McNab A. A. Reversal of floppy eyelid syndrome with treatment of obstructive sleep apnoea. *Clin. Experiment Ophthalmol.*, 2000; 28: 125–6.

[47] Hayirci E., Yagci A., Palamar M., et al. The effect of continuous positive airway pressure treatment for obstructive sleep apnea syndrome on the ocular surface *Cornea,* 2012; 31:604-8.

[48] Harrison W., Pence N., Kovacich S. Anterior segment complications secondary to continuous positive airway pressure machine treatment in patients with obstructive sleep apnea *Optometry,* 2007; 78:352-5.

In: Eye Diseases …
Editor: Mingwu Wang
ISBN: 978-1-63482-894-9

Chapter 4

Keratoconus and Obstructive Sleep Apnea

William Stevenson, MD and Mingwu Wang*, MD, PhD
Department of Ophthalmology and Vision Science,
University of Arizona College of Medicine, AZ, US

Case Presentation

A young obese man with a history of refractive error presents for an evaluation of blurry vision This is the third time in the past few years that he has been seen for blurry or distorted vision. At the last encounter, symptomatic improvement was obtained with a change in eyeglass prescription. The physician's manifest refraction reveals progressively increasing myopia and astigmatism Interestingly, a unique 'scissoring' of the red reflex is observed on retinoscopy. Slit-lamp biomicroscopy reveals subtle abnormalities in the endothelial specular reflection. These findings prompt further evaluation with corneal tomography that confirms the diagnosis of keratoconus.

* mwang@eyes.arizona.edu

Keratoconus: An Overview

The cornea is the transparent avascular tissue that covers the front of the eye. The cornea provides approximately two-thirds of the refractive power of the eye. Corneal ectasia denotes progressive thinning and steepening of the cornea. Keratoconus, the most common primary corneal ectasia, is characterized by central corneal thinning and protrusion that cause the cornea to adopt a conical shape. [1] Distorting the shape of the cornea in this manner alters its refractive characteristics, thereby causing visual impairment. Advanced cases of keratoconus can involve refractive error and corneal scarring that are not amendable to optical correction. Consequently, keratoconus is one of the most common indications for corneal transplantation. [2]

Keratoconus is the most common primary corneal degeneration in the United States of America. [3] The prevalence of keratoconus is thought to be about 0.05 percent in the United States of America. [4] However, a prevalence of 2.3 percent has been reported in central India, suggesting that keratoconus may be more common in those of Asian descent. [5, 6] Moreover, keratoconus tends to present at an earlier age and progress more rapidly in those of Indian ethnicity. [7] Conflicting findings have been published regarding the prevalence of keratoconus in males and females, and although there may be a slight male predominance, this has not been definitively determined. [8, 9]

Keratoconus is generally a bilateral condition; however, it frequently demonstrates asymmetric corneal involvement. [10, 11] Keratoconus typically starts developing during adolescence and manifests during the second or third decade of life, after which the progression eventually stops. Common presenting complaints include blurred vision, distorted vision, and needing to change glasses frequently. The severity of keratoconus can range from mild corneal astigmatism to severe corneal scarring. The clinical signs of keratoconus vary based on the condition's severity; for example, 'scissoring' of the red reflex on ophthalmoscopy or retinoscopy is an early sign of keratoconus, while a V-shaped protrusion of the lower eyelid on downgaze, known as *Munson's sign*, is a late sign of keratoconus (Figure 1). Advanced keratoconus can precipitate breaks in Descemet's membrane, thereby causing pain, photophobia, and corneal edema; this condition is known as corneal hydrops and frequently results in sight-threatening corneal scarring. Corneal tomography, an imaging technique that maps the curvatures of the cornea, can assist in the diagnosis of keratoconus (Figure 2). Tomographic findings suggestive of keratoconus include inferonasal or inferotemporal thinning and steepening. However, there is no universally accepted diagnostic criteria for keratoconus, so accurate diagnosis requires consideration of the entire clinical picture.

Keratoconus is a multifactorial disorder that involves genetic, behavioral, and environmental factors Most cases of keratoconus are sporadic; however, autosomal dominant, autosomal recessive, and complex inheritance patterns have been described. [12-14] Cases of keratoconus tend to cluster in first-degree relatives and monozygotic twins, and consanguinity is a risk factor for keratoconus. [4, 15, 16]

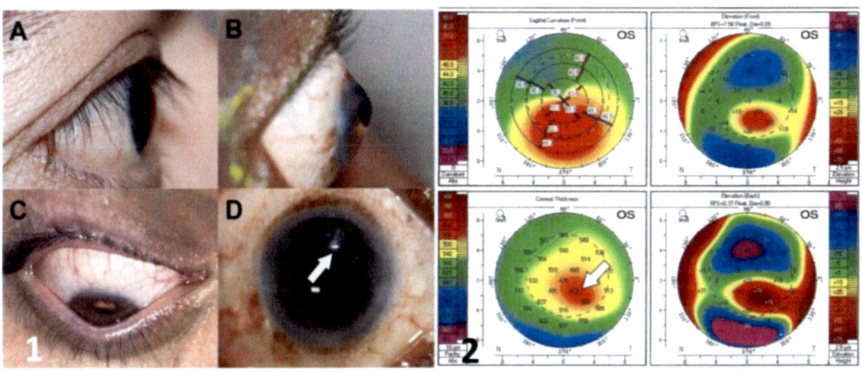

Figure 1. Color photographs of (A) a normal eye and (B) a keratoconic eye as viewed from the side. Color photograph (C) demonstrating *Munson's sign* – note the V-shaped protrusion of the lower eyelid on downgaze. Slit-lamp color photograph (D) showing a keratoconic eye as viewed from the front – note the white arrow delineating the decentered corneal apex (the most anterior point of the cornea when the eye is in primary position). Figure 2. A left eye corneal tomography of a keratoconic patient using Pentacam (Oculus, Wetzlar, Germany). The sagittal curvature map (top left) demonstrates inferior steepening of the cornea. The anterior and posterior elevation maps (top right and bottom right, respectively) demonstrate the magnitude of elevation (protrusion) of these corneal surfaces. The corneal thickness map (bottom left) demonstrates corneal thinning, with the thinnest point of the cornea (457μm) located slightly inferotemporal to the corneal center.

A variety of genes have been implicated in keratoconus; for example, the visual system homeobox 1 (VSX1) gene plays a role in ocular development and may account for a minority of keratoconus cases. [17, 18] Persistent eye rubbing, a behavior frequently observed in those with atopic disease, causes low-grade mechanical stress that may precipitate keratoconus. [19, 20] Ultraviolet light exposure is an environmental factor that may explain the increased prevalence of keratoconus in countries with warm, sunny climates. [21]

The clinical disorders associated with keratoconus are diverse, including but not limited to other corneal dystrophies (e.g., posterior polymorphous corneal dystrophy and Fuch's endothelial dystrophy) and ocular disorders (e.g., Leber's congenital amaurosis and tapetoretinal degeneration), atopic disorders (e.g., allergy and eczema), obstructive sleep apnea (OSA), connective tissue disorders (e.g., Marfan's syndrome and brittle cornea syndrome), chromosomal abnormalities (e.g., Down's syndrome and Turner's syndrome) and other genetic disorders (e.g., Williams syndrome and Costello syndrome). [19, 20, 22-31] Potential pathogenic etiologies of keratoconus include repetitive low-grade mechanical stress, oxidative damage, aberrant localized inflammation, and excess protease activity. [32-35] Regardless of the underlying etiology, morphologic changes of the cornea in keratoconus include thinning of the epithelium, fragmentation of Bowman's layer, thinning and scarring of the stroma, and folds or breaks in Descemet's membrane. [36]

The treatment of choice for keratoconus depends primarily on its degree of severity. Early keratoconus typically manifests as myopia or astigmatism that is amenable to optical correction with spectacles. However, cases of irregular astigmatism frequently require contact lenses. [37] Soft contact lenses can be effective in mild cases, while rigid gas-permeable lenses or more complex lens systems can be effective in moderate to severe cases. [38] Intracorneal ring segments, implantable collamer lenses, intraocular lenses, and refractive surgery have all been used to correct refractive error in cases of keratoconus. [39-42]. Corneal crosslinking with riboflavin and ultraviolet light has been shown to arrest the progression of corneal ectasia in some cases. [43] Cases of corneal hydrops may require symptomatic treatment with patching, bandage contact lenses, or medical therapy Refractory cases of keratoconus may necessitate corneal transplantation, such as deep anterior lamellar keratoplasty or penetrating keratoplasty, with generally favorable results. [44, 45]

Obstructive Sleep Apnea and Keratoconus

The keratoconus patients seen in clinical practice are disproportionately young, raising the question: where are the elderly keratoconus patients? [46, 47] Although this question has not been definitively answered, one potential explanation is that keratoconus is associated with numerous conditions that can cause early mortality, such as Down syndrome, mitral valve prolapse, and OSA. [48, 49] OSA is a particularly dangerous clinical etiology The recurrent episodes of hypoxia and reoxygenation caused by OSA result in sympathetic overactivity, inflammation, and coagulation. [50-52] OSA may play a causative role in numerous deleterious conditions including weight gain and obesity, hypertension, diabetes mellitus type 2, atherosclerosis, heart attack, stroke, and death. [51-58] Appropriate treatment of OSA (e.g., positive airway pressure) has been shown to reduce morbidity and mortality. The conditions associated with keratoconus extend beyond the eye and can be matters of life and death.

There is a surprisingly strong relationship between keratoconus and OSA. Corneal thinning is a central component of keratoconus, and corneal thinning has been described in OSA. [59] As the severity of OSA increases, central corneal thickness decreases; moreover, as minimum measured oxygen saturation decreases, central corneal thickness also decreases. There have been numerous studies investigating the prevalence of OSA in keratoconus. A majority of these studies have determined that keratoconus patients have a higher prevalence of OSA than healthy individuals, and the prevalence of OSA in keratoconus patients is reportedly as high as 24 percent. [49, 60, 61] Moreover, a striking number of keratoconus patients who do not have OSA are at high risk of developing OSA. [61]

Keratoconus and OSA are associated with several interlinked clinical conditions, namely obesity and floppy eyelid syndrome (FES). Obesity has been directly linked to keratoconus; keratoconus patients have an average body mass index of up to 32.4 and a prevalence of obesity of up to 52 percent. [60] Obesity is the most powerful risk factor for OSA, with a prevalence of obesity in OSA of approximately 70 percent. [62] Both obesity and OSA have been associated with FES, a condition characterized by laxity of the eyelids. [63, 64] Interestingly, keratoconus patients in general have been shown to have increased laxity of their eyelids similar to that seen in FES. [60] It is tempting to explain the association between OSA and keratoconus using these inter-related clinical conditions; for example, one might surmise that obesity induces OSA, obesity and OSA induce FES, and FES in turn induces keratoconus.

Keratoconus and OSA are complex disease entities. Numerous theories based on commonalities have been proposed to explain the connection between these disorders. Given that OSA induces repetitive episodes of hypoxia, it has been suggested that hypoxia and reperfusion injury may play a role in the development of keratoconus; however, there is little evidence to support this theory. [61] Both keratoconus and OSA have been associated with connective tissues disorders, such as Marfan's syndrome. [65] The pathogenesis of these conditions may involve connective tissue abnormalities that simultaneously weaken the cornea and upper airway; however, no single connective tissue abnormality has been described to link these conditions in a majority of cases.

Inflammation is one factor that may link keratoconus and OSA. Keratoconus has classically been considered a non-inflammatory condition; however, recent findings suggest that the pathogenesis of keratoconus may involve local inflammatory dysregulation. The tears of keratoconus patients have been shown to contain aberrant levels of various cytokines, including interleukin (IL)-6 and tumor necrosis factor (TNF)-α, as compared to the tears of healthy controls, suggesting that localized inflammation contributes to keratoconus. [34, 66] In OSA, there is evidence that recurrent collapse and expansion of the upper airway causes localized upper airway inflammation. [67] Furthermore, systemic inflammation plays a central role in the pathology of OSA. Recurrent episodes of hypoxic stress, such as those that occur in OSA, induce systemic inflammation characterized by the increased expression of a variety of cytokines (including IL-6 and TNF-α), chemokines, and cell adhesion molecules. [51] It remains to be seen if the systemic inflammation induced by OSA plays a role in the pathogenesis of select cases of keratoconus.

The abnormal expression of proteases and protease inhibitors has been described in both keratoconus and OSA. Given that keratoconus involves degradation of the extracellular matrix, protease activity has long been a subject of interest. Studies have demonstrated that keratoconus corneal cultures possess elevated collagenase activity, and an overall increase in the ratio of matrix metalloproteases (MMPs) to tissue inhibitor of matrix metalloproteinases (TIMPs) has been described. [68-70] The eyelids of patients with FES and the tears of patients with keratoconus patients contain elevated levels of MMP -9. [66, 71] Interestingly, the serum of patients with OSA has been found to contain elevated levels of MMP-9. [72] The increase of MMP-9 in OSA has been attributed to hypoxia-induced production of MMP-9 by monocytes. [73] Monocytes are known to migrate from the bloodstream into various tissues where they differentiate into resident macrophages and dendritic cell s, such as those found in the eyelid and cornea Whether or not the increased expression of proteases, such as MMP-9, in OSA plays a role in the development of FES or keratoconus remains to be seen.

Mechanical stress has long been recognized as a risk factor for the development of keratoconus Eye rubbing secondary to eye irritation has been reported in a majority of keratoconus patients, and intense eye rubbing has been linked to episodes of corneal hydrops. [74] OSA has been associated with signs and symptoms of dry eye disease that may lead to eye rubbing. [75] The treatment of OSA with positive airway pressure may actually increase ocular irritation, potentially through air-leakage around the mask; however, there is evidence that long-term treatment with appropriate positive airway pressure can alleviate ocular irritation. [76, 77] Sleep position may also play a role in the development of keratoconus. Some cases of OSA are positional in nature; these patients may sleep on their sides to limit snoring and decrease the frequency of apneic episodes. [49] Both keratoconus and FES have predilections to develop on the side of sleeping preference. Appropriate treatment with positive airway pressure can allow patients to return to their normal sleeping positions, potentially lessening the progression of keratoconus. Additionally, the eyelid may contribute to keratoconus through low-grade mechanical stress to the inferior cornea Trauma attributable to frequent episodes of eyelid eversion, such as that seen in FES, may contribute to the development of keratoconus, again highlighting the complex relationships between obesity, OSA, FES, and keratoconus. [63] The appropriate treatment of OSA is essential for decreasing patient morbidity and mortality In addition to improving overall health, the successful treatment of OSA may also improve ocular surface health. However, the effect of successful treatment of OSA on the development or progression of keratoconus remains unclear. Nevertheless, physicians and other healthcare professionals should be cognizant of the links between obesity, OSA, FES, and keratoconus. In patients with OSA, ocular complaints should be routinely solicited. Symptoms suggestive of keratoconus, such as blurred vision, distorted vision, and needing to change glasses frequently, should prompt referral to an eye care provider. It is equally important for eye care providers to remember that they play an integral role in recognizing and managing conditions that extend far beyond the eyes.

References

[1] Vazirani J, Basu S. Keratoconus: current perspectives. *Clin. Ophthalmol.* 2013;7:2019-30.

[2] Ghosheh FR, Cremona FA, Rapuano CJ, et al. Trends in penetrating keratoplasty in the United States 1980-2005. *Int. Ophthalmol.* 2008;28(3):147-53.

[3] National Eye Institute. Facts about the cornea and corneal disease. Available at: https://www.nei.nih.gov/health /cornealdisease. Accessed January 3, 2015.

[4] Kennedy RH, Bourne WM, Dyer JA. A 48-year clinical and epidemiologic study of keratoconus *Am. J. Ophthalmol* 1986;101(3):267-73.

[5] Pearson AR, Soneji B, Sarvananthan N, Sandforth-Smith JH. Does ethnic origin influence the incidence or severity of keratoconus? *Eye* (Lond) 2000;14:625–8.

[6] Jonas J.B, Nangia V, Matin A, et al. Prevalence and associations of keratoconus in rural Maharashtra in central India: The central India Eye Medical Study. *Am. J. Ophthalmol.* 2009;148:760–5.

[7] Saini JS, Saroha V, Singh P, et al. Keratoconus in Asian eyes at a tertiary eye care facility. *Clin. Exp. Optom.* 2004;87:97–101.

[8] Krachmer JH, Feder RS, Belin MW. Keratoconus and related non-inflammatory corneal thinning disorders. *Surv. Ophthalmol.* 1984;28:293–322.

[9] Wagner H, Barr JT, Zadnik K. Collaborative longitudinal evaluation of keratoconus (CLEK) study: Methods and findings to date. *Cont. Lens. Anterior Eye* 2007;30:223–32.

[10] Amsler M. Some data on the problem of keratoconus *Bull Sot Belge Ophthalmol.* 1961;129:331–54.

[11] Li X. Longitudinal study of the normal eyes in unilateral keratoconus patients. *Ophthalmology* 2004;111(3):440–446.

[12] Tyynismaa H, Sistonen P, Tuupanen S, et al. A locus for autosomal dominant keratoconus: linkage to 16q22.3-q23.1 in Finnish families *Invest. Ophthalmol Vis. Sci.* 2002;43(10):3160-4.

[13] Wang Y, Rabinowitz YS, Rotter JI, Yang H. Genetic epidemiological study of keratoconus: evidence for major gene determination. *Am. J. Med. Genet.* 2000;93(5):403-9.

[14] Burdon KP, Coster DJ, Charlesworth JC, et al. Apparent autosomal dominant keratoconus in a large Australian pedigree accounted for by digenic inheritance of two novel *loci Hum. Genet.* 2008;124(4):379-86.

[15] Tuft SJ, Hassan H, George S, et al. Keratoconus in 18 pairs of twins *Acta. Ophthalmol.* 2012;90(6):e482-6.

[16] Georgiou T, Funnell CL, Cassels-Brown A, O'Conor R. Influence of ethnic origin on the incidence of keratoconus and associated atopic disease in Asians and white patients. *Eye* (Lond) 2004;18(4):379-83.

[17] Bisceglia L, De Bonis P, Pizzicoli C, et al. Linkage analysis in keratoconus: replication of locus 5q21.2 and identification of other suggestive Loci. *Invest. Ophthalmol. Vis. Sci.* 2009;50(3):1081-6.

[18] Héon E, Greenberg A, Kopp KK, et al. VSX1: a gene for posterior polymorphous dystrophy and keratoconus *Hum. Mol. Genet.* 2002;11(9):1029-36.

[19] McMonnies CW, Boneham GC. Keratoconus, allergy, itch, eye-rubbing and hand-dominance *Clin. Exp. Optom* 2003;86(6):376-84.

[20] Bawazeer AM, Hodge WG, Lorimer B. Atopy and keratoconus: a multivariate analysis *Br. J. Ophthalmol.* 2000;84(8):834-6.

[21] Wojcik KA, Kaminska A, Blasiak J, et al. Oxidative stress in the pathogenesis of keratoconus and Fuchs endothelial corneal dystrophy *Int. J. Mol. Sci.* 2013;14(9):19294-308.

[22] Lechner J, Dash DP, Muszynska D, et al. Mutational spectrum of the ZEB1 gene in corneal dystrophies supports a genotype-phenotype correlation *Invest Ophthalmol. Vis. Sci.* 2013;54(5):3215-23.

[23] Lipman RM, Rubenstein JB, Torczynski E. Keratoconus and Fuchs' corneal endothelial dystrophy in a patient and her family. *Arch. Ophthalmol.* 1990;108(7):993-4.

[24] Elder MJ. Leber congenital amaurosis and its association with keratoconus and keratoglobus. *J. Pediatr. Ophthalmol. Strabismus* 1994;31(1):38-40.

[25] Moschos M, Droutsas D, Panagakis E, et al. Keratoconus and tapetoretinal degeneration. *Cornea* 1996;15(5):473-6.

[26] Bass HN, Sparkes RS, Crandall BF, Marcy SM. Congenital contractural arachnodactyly, keratoconus, and probable Marfan syndrome in the same pedigree *J. Pediatr* 1981;98(4):591-3.

[27] Al-Hussain H, Zeisberger SM, Huber PR, et al. Brittle cornea syndrome and its delineation from the kyphoscoliotic type of Ehlers-Danlos syndrome (EDS VI): report on 23 patients and review of the literature. *Am. J. Med. Genet. A* 2004;124A(1):28-34.

[28] Vincent AL, Weiser BA, Cupryn M, et al. Computerized corneal topography in a paediatric population with Down syndrome *Clin. Experiment. Ophthalmol.* 2005;33(1):47-52.

[29] Macsai M, Maguen E, Nucci P. Keratoconus and Turner's syndrome Cornea 1997;16(5):534-6.

[30] Viana MM, Frasson M, Leão LL, et al. A new case of keratoconus associated with Williams-Beuren syndrome *Ophthalmic. Genet.* 2013;34(3):174-7.

[31] Gripp KW, Demmer LA. Keratoconus in Costello syndrome *Am. J. Med. Genet. A* 2013;161A(5):1132-6.

[32] McMonnies CW. Mechanisms of rubbing-related corneal trauma in keratoconus *Cornea* 2009;28(6):607-15.

[33] Kenney MC, Chwa M, Atilano SR, et al. Increased levels of catalase and cathepsin V/L2 but decreased TIMP-1 in keratoconus corneas: evidence that oxidative stress plays a role in this disorder *Invest. Ophthalmol. Vis. Sci.* 2005;46(3):823-32.

[34] Jun AS, Cope L, Speck C, et al. Subnormal cytokine profile in the tear fluid of keratoconus patients. *PLoS One* 2011;6(1):e16437.

[35] Zhou L, Sawaguchi S, Twining SS, et al. Expression of degradative enzymes and protease inhibitors in corneas with keratoconus *Invest. Ophthalmol. Vis. Sci.* 1998;39(7):1117-24.

[36] Sherwin T, Brookes NH. Morphological changes in keratoconus: pathology or pathogenesis *Clin Experiment Ophthalmol.* 2004;32(2): 211–217.

[37] Weed KH, MacEwen CJ, McGhee CN. The Dundee University Scottish Keratoconus Study II: a prospective study of optical and surgical correction. *Ophthalmic. Physiol. Opt.* 2007;27(6):561–567.

[38] Barnett M, Mannis MJ. Contact lenses in the management of keratoconus *Cornea* 2011;30(12):1510–1516.

[39] Colin J, Cochener B, Savary G, Malet F. Correcting keratoconus with intracorneal rings *J. Cataract. Refract. Surg.* 2000;26(8):1117-22.

[40] Kamiya K, Shimizu K, Ando W, et al. Phakic toric implantable collamer lens implantation for the correction of high myopic astigmatism in eyes with keratoconus *J. Refract. Surg.* 2008;24(8): 840–842.

[41] Thebpatiphat N, Hammersmith KM, Rapuano CJ, et al. Cataract surgery in keratoconus *Eye Contact Lens* 2007;33(5):244–246.

[42] Bilgihan K, Ozdek SC, Konuk O, et al. Results of photorefractive keratectomy in keratoconus suspects at 4 years. *J. Refract. Surg.* 2000;16(4):438–443.

[43] Wollensak G, Spoerl E, Seiler T. Riboflavin/ultraviolet-A-induced collagen crosslinking for the treatment of keratoconus *Am. J. Ophthalmol.* 2003;135(5):620–627.

[44] Sarnicola V, Toro P, Gentile D, Hannush SB. Descemetic DALK and predescemetic DALK: outcomes in 236 cases of keratoconus *Cornea* 2010;29(1):53–59.

[45] Javadi MA, Motlagh BF, Jafarinasab MR, et al. Outcomes of penetrating keratoplasty in keratoconus *Cornea* 2005;24(8):941–946.

[46] Ertan A, Muftuoglu O. Keratoconus clinical findings according to different age and gender groups. *Cornea* 2008;27(10):1109-13.

[47] McMonnies CW. Where are the older keratoconus patients? *Cornea* 2009;28(7):836.

[48] Lichter H, Loya N, Sagie A, Cohen N. Keratoconus and mitral valve prolapse *Am. J. Ophthalmol.* 2000;129(5):667–668.

[49] Gupta PK, Stinnett SS, Carlson AN. Prevalence of sleep apnea in patients with keratoconus *Cornea* 2012;31(6):595-9.

[50] Imadojemu VA, Mawji Z, Kunselman A, et al. Sympathetic chemoreflex responses in obstructive sleep apnea and effects of continuous positive airway pressure therapy *Chest* 2007;131(5):1406-13.

[51] Nadeem R, Molnar J, Madbouly EM, et al. Serum inflammatory markers in obstructive sleep apnea: a meta-analysis *J. Clin. Sleep. Med.* 2013;9(10):1003-12.

[52] Toraldo DM, Peverini F, De Benedetto M, De Nuccio F. Obstructive sleep apnea syndrome: blood viscosity, blood coagulation abnormalities, and early atherosclerosis *Lung* 2013;191(1):1-7.

[53] Phillips BG, Kato M, Narkiewicz K, et al. Increases in leptin levels, sympathetic drive, and weight gain in obstructive sleep apnea *Am. J. Physiol. Heart Circ. Physiol.* 2000;279(1):H234–H237.

[54] Pepperell JC, Ramdassingh-Dow S, Crosthwaite N, et al. Ambulatory blood pressure after therapeutic and subtherapeutic nasal continuous positive airway pressure for obstructive sleep apnoea: a randomised parallel trial *Lancet* 2002;359(9302):204–210.

[55] Lévy P, Pépin JL, Arnaud C, et al. Obstructive sleep apnea and atherosclerosis *Prog. Cardiovasc. Dis.* 2009;51(5):400-10.

[56] Punjabi NM, Shahar E, Redline S, et al. Sleep-disordered breathing, glucose intolerance, and insulin resistance: the Sleep Heart Health Study. *Am. J. Epidemiol.* 2004;160(6):521-30.

[57] Marin JM, Carrizo SJ, Vicente E, Agusti AG. Long-term cardiovascular outcomes in men with obstructive sleep apnoea-hypopnoea with or without treatment with continuous positive airway pressure: an observational study. *Lancet* 2005;365(9464):1046-53.

[58] Yaggi HK, Concato J, Kernan WN, et al. Obstructive sleep apnea as a risk factor for stroke and death. *N. Engl. J. Med.* 2005;353(19):2034-41.

[59] Ekinci M, Huseyinoglu N, Cagatay HH, et al. Is there a relationship between sleep apnea and central corneal thickness? *Curr. Eye Res.* 2013;38(11):1104-9.

[60] Pihlblad MS, Schaefer DP. Eyelid laxity, obesity, and obstructive sleep apnea in keratoconus *Cornea* 2013;32(9):1232-6.

[61] Saidel MA, Paik JY, Garcia C, et al. Prevalence of sleep apnea syndrome and high-risk characteristics among keratoconus patients. *Cornea* 2012;31(6):600-3.

[62] Malhotra A, White DP. Obstructive sleep apnoea. *Lancet* 2002;360(9328):237-45.

[63] Fowler AM, Dutton JJ. Floppy eyelid syndrome as a subset of lax eyelid conditions: relationships and clinical relevance (an ASOPRS thesis). *Ophthal. Plast. Reconstr. Surg.* 2010;26(3):195-204.

[64] Ezra DG, Beaconsfield M, Sira M, et al. The associations of floppy eyelid syndrome: a case control study. *Ophthalmology* 2010;117(4):831-8.

[65] Cistulli PA, Sullivan CE. Sleep apnea in Marfan's syndrome Increased upper airway collapsibility during sleep *Chest* 1995;108(3):631-5.

[66] Lema I, Durán JA. Inflammatory molecules in the tears of patients with keratoconus *Ophthalmology* 2005;112(4):654-9.

[67] Almendros I, Carreras A, Ramírez J, et al. Upper airway collapse and reopening induce inflammation in a sleep apnoea model. *Eur. Respir. J.* 2008;32(2):399-404.

[68] Kao WW, Vergnes JP, Ebert J, et al. Increased collagenase and gelatinase activities in keratoconus *Biochem. Biophys. Res. Commun.* 1982;107:929–936.

[69] Rehany U, Lahav M, Shoshan S. Collagenolytic activity in keratoconus *Ann. Ophthalmol.* 1982;14:751–754.

[70] Kenney MC, Chwa M, Opbroek AJ, et al. Increased gelatinolytic activity in keratoconus keratocyte cultures. A correlation to an altered matrix metalloproteinase -2/tissue inhibitor of metalloproteinase ratio. *Cornea* 1994;13:114–124

[71] Schlötzer-Schrehardt U, Stojkovic M, Hofmann-Rummelt C, et al. The pathogenesis of floppy eyelid syndrome: involvement of matrix metalloproteinases in elastic fiber degradation *Ophthalmology* 2005;112(4):694-704.

[72] Tazaki T, Minoguchi K, Yokoe T, et al. Increased levels and activity of matrix metalloproteinase -9 in obstructive sleep apnea syndrome *Am. J. Respir. Crit. Care. Med.* 2004;170(12):1354-9.

[73] Tamaki S' Yamauchi M, Fukuoka A, et al. Production of inflammatory mediators by monocytes in patients with obstructive sleep apnea syndrome *Intern. Med.* 2009;48(15):1255-62.

[74] Zadnik K, Barr JT, Edrington TB, et al. Baseline findings in the Collaborative Longitudinal Evaluation of Keratoconus (CLEK) Study. *Invest. Ophthalmol. Vis. Sci.* 1998;39(13):2537-46.

[75] Acar M, Firat H, Acar U, Ardic S. Ocular surface assessment in patients with obstructive sleep apnea-hypopnea syndrome *Sleep Breath* 2013;17(2):583-8.

[76] Hayirci E, Yagci A, Palamar M, et al. The effect of continuous positive airway pressure treatment for obstructive sleep apnea syndrome on the ocular surface *Cornea* 2012;31(6):604-8.

[77] Acar M, Firat H, Yuceege M, Ardic S. Long-term effects of PAP on ocular surface in obstructive sleep apnea syndrome *Can. J. Ophthalmol.* 2014;49(2):217-21.

In: Eye Diseases ...
Editor: Mingwu Wang

ISBN: 978-1-63482-894-9

Chapter 5

Retinal Vein Occlusion and Obstructive Sleep Apnea

Lauren Imbornoni, MD, Mingwu Wang, MD, PhD and John Christoforidis*, MD
Department of Ophthalmology and Vision Science,
University of Arizona College of Medicine, AZ, US

Case Presentation

A 67-year old African American female with history of hypertension, type II diabetes mellitus and obstructive sleep apnea presents to the eye clinic with sudden vision loss in the left eye that she discovered upon awakening. She denies eye pain, eye redness, photophobia and flashes of light She has no past ocular history. She takes lisinopril and metformin, and uses a continuous positive airway pressure machine at night. On examination, best corrected visual acuity in the right eye is 20/20 and in the left eye, 20/400. Pupil exam reveals a relative afferent pupillary defect in the left eye. Intraocular pressure is normal in both eyes by applanation tonometry Slit lamp examination shows normal anterior segments with open angles bilaterally. Fundoscopic exam of the right eye reveals a cup-to-disk ratio of 0.4 with sharp rim and flat macula.

* Email: jchristoforidis@eyes.arizona.edu

Fundoscopic exam of the left eye reveals optic nerve edema, as well as diffuse retinal hemorrhages in all four quadrants of the foundus and dilated, tortuous retinal veins (Figure 1). The presentation and exam findings in this patient are consistent with central retinal vein occlusion.

Retinal Vein Occlusion: An Overview

Retinal vein occlusion (RVO) is the second most common retinal vascular disease after diabetic retinopathy and a significant cause of visual loss in adults. [1-3] RVO occurs when a retinal vein becomes obstructed, which interrupts the normal venous drainage of retinal tissue This leads to hemorrhage and edema of the retina corresponding to the area of distribution of the occluded vein and can cause immediate vision loss. Potential visual-threatening complications include the formation of macular edema, neovascularization, vitreous hemorrhage, and neovascular glaucoma. [3] RVO is classically linked to systemic disorders including hypertension, diabetes mellitus and cardiovascular disease, and ocular conditions such as glaucoma. [3] It has recently been linked to obstructive sleep apnea (OSA). [4, 5] RVO and OSA are likely connected through shared comorbid conditions, including hypertension and diabetes mellitus. However, the relationship may be more complex, and it is thought that the systemic and local changes seen in people with OSA directly contribute to the pathogenesis of RVO.

RVO is classified by the location of the occlusion; either the central retinal vein or one of its branches can become occluded. Central retinal vein occlusion (CRVO) occurs due to a blockage that is most likely at the level of the lamina cribrosa of the optic nerve and affects all four quadrants of the retina Branch retinal vein occlusion (BRVO) occurs when a branch of the central retinal vein becomes occluded, affecting a smaller portion of the retinal tissue. [3] A third pattern of occlusion is a hemiretinal vein occlusion (HRVO), which occurs when the venous outflow at the proximal portion of the branches emanating from the central retinal vein is occluded and the superior or inferior retina is subsequently impaired. There is no consensus as to whether HRVO is a variant of BRVO or CRVO. [3] However, this type of occlusion is much less common, and most literature regarding RVOs focuses on CRVO and BRVO.

CRVO is more severe, but less common than BRVO. CRVO is estimated to affect 2.5 million adults worldwide, while BRVO is estimated to affect 13.9

million. [6] The prevalence of BRVO ranges between 0.4% and 0.6%, [6, 7] and that of CRVO between 0.08% and 0.1%. [6, 7] The Prevalence of both CRVO and BRVO increases with increasing age. [6]

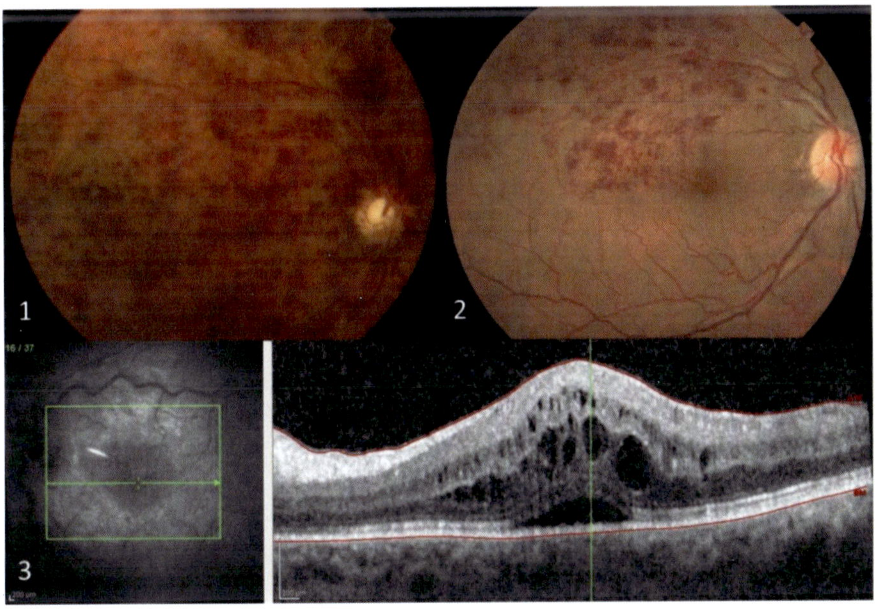

Figure 1. Color fundus photograph of a right eye in a patient with central retinal vein occlusion demonstrating optic nerve edema, tortuous venules and profound intraretinal hemorrhages in all 4 quadrants of the fundus and throughout the macula. Figure 2. Color fundus photograph of a right eye in a patient with a superior branch retinal vein occlusion demonstrating arteriolar sclerosis with arteriovenous nicking. The area of blockage is at the proximal portion of the superior temporal arcade with intraretinal hemorrhages and few exudates present distally. Figure 3. Spectral domain optical coherence tomography with Heidelberg Spectralis® demonstrating the presence of cystoid macular edema and subretinal fluid in a patient with central retinal vein occlusion of the left eye.

Their prevalence by gender. [1, 2, 6, 8, 9] RVO was found to be more prevalent in those of Asian and Hispanic descents, [6] although, in a different analysis, RVO was found to be more prevalent in those of black race when compared to non-Hispanic whites. [9, 10]

CRVO presents as sudden, painless, unilateral loss of vision The presentation of BRVO is variable and depends on the location and severity of the occlusion BRVO may be asymptomatic, or it may present with visual field deficit corresponding to the involved retinal region. [3] Fundoscopic exam in

RVO characteristically reveals intraretinal hemorrhages, as well as dilated and tortuous retinal veins. In CRVO, there are diffuse hemorrhages in all four quadrants giving the distinctive "blood and thunder" appearance (Figure 1). In BRVO, the hemorrhages are focal, localized to one retinal quadrant, and appear along the distribution of the affected retinal vein (Figure 2). Cotton-wool spots and macular edema may occur in both types. Retinal neovascularization is seen almost exclusively with BRVO, and optic nerve edema is more prevalent with CRVO. [11] Fluorescein angiography is typically performed to assess the presence of retinal neovascularization and macular edema, and to quantify the amount of retinal non-perfusion. [12] Optical coherence tomography is a diagnostic tool that identifies and quantifies the presence of macular edema in both conditions (Figure 3). [3, 11]

The mechanism of occlusion differs between CRVO and BRVO. CRVO occurs due to thrombus formation within the lumen of the central retinal vein at, or posterior to, the lamina cribrosa. [3] Thrombus formation is thought to occur due to compression from the adjacent central retinal artery within the shared adventitial sheath. Arterial disease, such as atherosclerosis, causes the central retinal artery to become rigid and sclerotic, which can compress the adjacent vein, cause turbulent blood flow, and secondarily induce thrombus formation within the lumen of the vein. [3, 9, 11] Pathogenesis of CRVO in younger adults without cardiovascular risk factors differs from older adults with atherosclerosis. It was found that individuals 45 years of age and younger who develop RVO have a high prevalence of coagulation disorders. [13]

In contrast, BRVO occurs at sites of arteriovenous crossing where a branch retinal artery crosses over a branch retinal vein within a shared adventitial sheath. [3, 8, 11, 14] Chronic systemic diseases, such as hypertension and diabetes mellitus, can damage the small retinal arterioles and lead arteriolar wall thickening, loss of elasticity, and rigidity of the vessel. As in CRVO, the damaged arteriole compresses the branch retinal vein, narrowing the lumen and damaging the endothelium of the vein. It is thought that this mechanical compression is the primary cause of occlusion in BRVO. [3, 11] BRVO can also result from thrombus formation, [3, 15] as in CRVO; however, compression alone is the most commonly cited mechanism of occlusion. [16]

Differences in risk factors for CRVO and BRVO support the proposed differences in pathogenesis Hypertension and glaucoma are consistently identified as risk factors for all RVOs. [9, 10] However, associations between RVO and diabetes, hyperlipidemia and hypercoagulable states are variable between studies. [10] Two large studies from the University of Michigan published in 2013 and 2014 identified risk factors specific to BRVO and CRVO, and clarified areas of inconsistency within the literature. [9, 10]

Atherosclerosis is thought to be a primary contributing factor to RVO. Markers for atherosclerosis were found to significantly increase the risk of RVO. Prior cerebrovascular accident increased the risk of CRVO by 45% and that of BRVO by 34%. [9, 10] Peripheral artery disease increased the risk for CRVO by 16%. [9, 10] Interestingly, dyslipidemia, a known risk factor of atherosclerosis, was not a significant risk factor for either BRVO or CRVO. A possible explanation is that arterial damage may depend on the severity and duration of atherosclerosis, and the vessels may not become rigid until late in the disease. It is also possible that treatment for dyslipidemia could confound the association. [9, 10]

Consistent with other reports, hypertension was a significant risk factor for CRVO and BRVO. Hypertension without end-organ damage increased the risk of CRVO and BRVO by 36%. [9, 10] Those with hypertension and end-organ damage had a 92% increased risk of CRVO and 107% increased risk of BRVO. [9. 10] Diabetes mellitus has been inconsistently associated with RVO. The variable results may be explained by separating DM with and without end organ damage. Diabetes without end-organ damage causes no increased risk of BRVO or CRVO. In contrast, DM with end-organ damage increased risk of CRVO by 53% and that of BRVO by 36%. [9, 10]

An important distinction between BRVO and CRVO was the risk associated with hypercoagulable state Hypercoagulable state increased the risk of CRVO by 145% but did not significantly increase the risk of BRVO. [9, 10] Virchow's triad describes three factors that predispose to thrombosis: endothelial damage, abnormal blood flow, and hypercoagulable state. Endothelial damage can be caused by diabetes and hypertension, and abnormal blood flow can result from atherosclerosis, which is also related to diabetes and hypertension. It is proposed that all three components of Virchow's triad increase the risk of CRVO, while the first two components are the most significant risk factors for BRVO. [9] This supports the difference in mechanism between the two, as CRVO most likely results from thrombus formation, while BRVO is most likely caused by mechanical compression associated with atherosclerosis. [9, 10]

In most cases, RVO causes immediate visual consequences and creates an ongoing risk of neovascularization Neovascularization can be located on the iris, anterior chamber angle, or retina, and can lead to vitreous hemorrhage and neovascular glaucoma. [3] In patients with RVO, the presenting visual acuity usually ranges from 20/40 to less than 20/200. [17, 18] Without treatment, visual acuity improves in 33% of eyes with BRVO, but stays reduced in most eyes with CRVO. [17, 18] Of those that do improve without treatment, improvement to better than 20/40 is very rare. [17, 18] RVO in one eye significantly increases the risk of RVO in the fellow eye. Of individuals with BRVO in one eye, 10% developed bilateral BRVO over time. [18] Five percent of individuals with CRVO developed another RVO in the fellow eye over a one year period. [17]

Treatment options for RVO are evolving. In the pre-anti-vascular endothelial growth factor (VEGF) era, laser photocoagulation treatment in a grid pattern for associated macular edema was found to be helpful for BRVO but not for CRVO. In addition, several reports explored surgical options toward the occluded vein as treatment for CRVO and BRVO. The techniques included lamina puncture, which creates an incision in the optic nerve head adjacent to the central retinal vein to create perivascular space and establish reperfusion, [19] and radial optic neurotomy, in which an incision at the nasal edge of the optic nerve head extends to the adjacent sclera to relieve pressure on the central retinal vein. [20, 21] Surgical decompression of BRVO was attempted via sheathotomy at the arteriovenous crossing with some success. [22] Injection of tissue plasminogen activator into occluded central [23] and branch [24] retinal veins was also explored as a treatment option, but found to cause significant adverse effects. [3] Surgical and thrombolytic approaches have fallen by the wayside as anti-VEGF therapy has gained favor.

Currently, management of RVO is primarily aimed at controlling their complications CRVO and BRVO without complications are simply observed. The mainstay treatment for macular edema associated with CRVO or BRVO is intravitreal therapy with anti-VEGF agents. The use of ranibizumab for RVO with macular edema was shown to achieve significant visual gains in two large clinical trials. [25] In eyes that develop neovascularization, the treatment for CRVO is panretinal photocoagulation, usually augmented with intravitreal anti-VEGF therapy, and for BRVO, is peripheral scattered laser photocoagulation with or without anti-VEGF therapy. [3, 15, 25, 26]

Retinal Vein Occlusion and Obstructive Sleep Apnea

RVO can cause significant and permanent ocular morbidity It arises from a combination of arterial disease and venous disease. Known systemic risk factors include hypertension, complicated forms of diabetes mellitus, stroke and hypercoagulable state Treatment is often challenging and individuals with RVO have significant risk of developing RVO in the fellow eye, which in severe cases, can cause blindness It is important to prevent RVO by identifying those at increased risk and taking measures to modify the risk factors Recently, OSA, a disorder characterized by episodes of complete or partial upper airway obstruction during sleep, [27] has been linked to the development of RVO. The pathophysiology of OSA may directly promote the formation of RVO.

The association between RVO and OSA was first described in 2009 by Leroux et al. [28]. They reported three patients who presented with RVO without conventional risk factors They were subsequently tested and found to all have OSA. The authors proposed that OSA could be a risk factor for the occurrence or aggravation of RVO. [28] The following year, this group published another study, with a series of 63 patients with RVO. [4] Of these patients, they identified a subset of 30 who had risk factors for OSA. They found OSA in 77% of this subset, a significantly higher prevalence than the estimated 2-7% in the general population. [4] Of the 30 individuals, 23 had CRVO, 5 had BRVO and 2 had HRVO. There was no significant difference found on the types of RVO. Although not all patients were screened for OSA, even if the remaining patients were and found negative, the prevalence of OSA in this series would still be 37%. This study shows OSA as a risk factor for RVO and in addition, poses the question of whether it could also be a triggering factor for RVO, as many patients with RVO discover vision loss upon awakening. [4] In 2011, this group published a prospective observational study of 61 individuals with RVO and found that vision loss was discovered upon awakening in 77% of patients with CRVO and 33% with BRVO. [29] Whether or not sleep disorders are a triggering factor for RVO remains to be seen.

The biggest study to date regarding the relationship between RVO and OSA was published in 2012 by Chou et al. [5] This was a nationwide, population-based retrospective, matched-control cohort study from Taiwan The study identified 5,965 individuals with newly diagnosed sleep apnea and recorded incidence of RVO over a mean of 3.72 years. It did not differentiate between OSA and central sleep apnea The sleep apnea cohort was compared to a control group of 29,669 individuals. During the study period, 13 individuals (0.22%) from the sleep apnea cohort developed BRVO and none developed CRVO. From the control group, 39 individuals (0.13%) developed RVO; 29 were BRVO and 10 were CRVO. Overall, patients with sleep apnea experienced a 1.94-fold increase in incident RVO, independent of gender, age and comorbidities. [5] It concluded that sleep apnea is independently associated with the development of RVO and hence an independent risk factor for RVO. This study has limitations. It assessed RVO as a whole, without differentiating between CRVO and BRVO. It is possible that sleep apnea may affect these disorders differently. Additionally, it did not differentiate between OSA and central sleep apnea; however, OSA accounts for 90% of sleep apnea in this population. Lastly, all subjects are of Chinese ethnicity and the results may not be generalizable to other ethnic groups. [5]

It is unclear how OSA contributes to the development of RVO as an independent risk factor. One proposed mechanism is through interconnected comorbidities. The established risk factors for OSA include overweight, obesity, and craniofacial abnormalities. [27, 30] However, these are not common risk factors for RVO, and would not necessarily put a person at increased risk for RVO. However, once an individual develops OSA, his risk for developing these comorbid conditions increases. OSA independently increases the risk of heart failure, coronary artery disease, hypertension, insulin resistance and type 2 diabetes mellitus. [31, 32, 33] Therefore, OSA may indirectly increase the risk of RVO through the promotion of comorbid conditions that are strong risk factors for RVO.

In addition to linked comorbidities, the local and systemic changes in OSA patients may directly impact the development of RVO. Intermittent episodes of hypoxia and hypercapnea from airway obstruction may locally affect the retinal microcirculation The hypoxia and hypercapnea are thought to induce vasodilation of the central retinal artery, which can cause compression of the adjacent central retinal vein and its tributaries within the shared adventitial sheath. This compression may alter hemodynamics and cause damage within the vessel. [4, 5] Additionally, hypercapnea is thought to induce cerebral vasodilation, which increases intracranial pressure and cerebrospinal fluid pressure. This may result in papilledema and increased venous pressure in the optic nerve head. [4, 5]

The combination of increased pressure and venous compression may slow the blood flow through the retina This could cause blood plasma to leak through the blood vessel wall, leading to a local increase in hematocrit and local hyperviscosity within the retinal vein. [4, 5] Additionally, frequent arousal from sleep in OSA activates the sympathetic nervous system, which leads to repetitive hemodynamic changes within the retinal vascular system. [4] These factors together promote vessel damage, stasis, thrombogenesis, and ultimately occlusion.

In addition to the local effects, OSA has systemic consequences that may promote RVO. The repeated episodes of hypoxia in OSA patients result in hypercoagulability, [34, 35] increased sympathetic activation, [27, 32, 35] increased platelet aggregability, [35] increased blood viscosity, [35] systemic inflammation, [32, 36, 37] oxidative stress, [32] and endothelial dysfunction [38] These factors contribute to all three components of Virchow's triad: endothelial dysfunction, abnormal blood flow and hypercoagulability, which lead to thrombosis.

The endothelial cell layer of blood vessels maintains vascular tone, mediates hemostasis and regulates inflammation Endothelial dysfunction is caused by, and contributes to hypertension and diabetes, both of which are promoted by OSA. [9] Endothelial dysfunction also promotes atherosclerosis OSA was found to directly contribute to endothelial dysfunction, independent of conventional risk factors. [38] Additionally, OSA increases reactive oxygen species, which impair endothelial function. [32] Endothelial dysfunction is related to abnormal blood flow, the second component of Virchow's triad. Abnormal blood flow is usually the result of venous stasis or turbulent flow secondary to atherosclerosis. [9] OSA promotes hypertension and diabetes, both of which contribute to atherosclerosis. [9] Additionally, OSA causes increased blood viscosity which can lead to stasis. [39]

There are several ways in which OSA contributes to the third component of Virchow's triad, hypercoagulability. Chronic hypoxemia leads to increased hematocrit levels, which can increase blood viscosity. [34, 35] Individuals with OSA are found to have increased platelet aggregability and activation, [35] as well as increased clotting factors, specifically factors XIIa, VIIa, thrombin-antithrombin (TAT), and soluble P-selectin (sP-sel). [40] Recurrent sympathetic activation at night increases catecholamines in the circulation, which can also stimulate platelet activity. [35, 39] Clotting factors and platelet activation act conjointly to promote a thrombogenic state in OSA patients.

Additionally, inflammation plays a key role in promoting a thrombogenic state Chronic systemic inflammation is characteristic of OSA and is caused, in part, by hypoxia and increased sympathetic activity. [5] Inflammatory cytokines, specifically C-reactive protein (CRP), tumor necrosis factor -α, and interleukin-6 levels are elevated in OSA patients, [36, 37] and may lead to coagulation and platelet aggregation CRP was specifically found to activate plasminogen activator inhibitor -1, which decreases the activity of plasminogen and fibrinolysis, preventing breakdown of clots. [5, 39] The inflammatory cytokines were found to cause the release of tissue factor from endothelial cells, which trigger the coagulation pathway, promoting clot formation [5] They were also found to decrease the levels of activated protein C, which ultimately increases the duration of the hypercoagulable state. [5] Lastly, the inflammatory cytokines are thought to release von Willebrand factor from the endothelial cells, promoting platelet aggregation.

OSA directly and indirectly promotes all three components of Virchow's triad and predisposes to thrombosis Perhaps it is through these systemic and local effects, OSA contributes to the development of RVO. There has been only a small number of studies exploring this relationship. [4, 5, 28, 29, 39] The studies linking RVO and OSA do not differentiate between CRVO and BRVO, which appear to have distinct risk factors, pathogenesis and prognosis It is likely that OSA contributes to the development of CRVO and BRVO in different ways. Based on the identified risk factors, all three components of Virchow's triad contribute to CRVO formation, while endothelial dysfunction and abnormal blood flow play the biggest role in BRVO development. [9] Further studies are needed to clarify the pathogenesis of RVO and improve the understanding of how specific risk factors contribute to RVO development.

RVO is a vision-threatening disorder with a complicated pathogenesis and evolving treatment options. Identifying those at increased risk and working to modify risk factors may decrease the burden of this disease. OSA was found in one large retrospective cohort study to independently contribute to RVO development. [5] Identifying those at increased risk for RVO will allow for the opportunity to modify specific risk factors. It is also important for clinicians to be aware of the association between RVO and OSA, as the diagnosis of RVO in an individual may prompt the clinician to evaluate for OSA. It is not yet known if treating OSA can decrease the risk, severity or prognosis of RVO. However, treatment of OSA can improve blood pressure and other components of the metabolic syndrome, which in turn, lower the risk for developing RVO [32].

References

[1] Mitchell P, Smith W, Chang A. Prevalence and associations of retinal vein occlusion in Australia. *Arch. Ophthalmol.* 1996;114:1243-7.

[2] Cugati S, Wang JJ, Rochtchina E, et al. Ten-year incidence of retinal vein occlusion in an older population: the blue mountains eye study. *Arch. Ophthalmol.* 2006;124:726-32.

[3] Ehlers JP, Fekrat S. Retinal vein occlusion: beyond the acute event. *Surv. Ophthalmol.* 2011;56:281-99.

[4] Glacet-Bernard A, Leroux les Jardins G, Lasry S, et al. Obstructive sleep apnea among patients with retinal vein occlusion *Arch. Ophthalmol.* 2010;128:1533-8.

[5] Chou KT, Huang CC, Tsai DC, et al. Sleep apnea and risk of retinal vascular occlusion: a nationwide population-based study of Taiwanese. *Am. J. Ophthalmol.* 2012;154:200-5.

[6] Rogers S, McIntosh RL, Journ BGD, et al. The prevalence of retinal vein occlusion: pooled data from population studies from the United States, Europe, Asia, and Australia. *Ophthalmology* 2010;117:313-9.

[7] Klein R, Klein BEK, Moss SE, et al. The epidemiology of retinal vein occlusion: the beaver dam eye study. *Tr. Am. Ophth. Soc.* 2000;98:133-43.

[8] Zhou JQ, Xu L, Wang S, et al. The 10-year incidence and risk factors of retinal vein occlusion: the Beijing eye study. *Ophthalmology* 2013;120:803-8.

[9] Newman-Casey PA, Stem M, Talwar N, et al. Risk factors associated with developing branch retinal vein occlusion among enrollees in a United States Managed Care Plan. *Ophthalmology* 2014;121:1939-48.

[10] Stem MS, Talwar N, Comer GM, et al. A longitudinal analysis of risk factors associated with central retinal vein occlusion s. *Ophthalmology* 2013;120:362-70.

[11] Jaulim A, Ahmed B, Khanam T, et al. Branch retinal vein occlusion: epidemiology, pathogenesis, risk factors, clinical features, diagnosis, and complications A update of the literature. *Retina* 2013;33:901-10.

[12] Baseline and early natural history report. The central vein occlusion study. *Arch. Ophthalmol.* 1993;111:1087-95.

[13] Kuhli-Hattenbach C, Scharrer I, Luchtenberg M, et al. Coagulation disorders and the risk of retinal vein occlusion *Thromb Haemost* 2010;103:299-305.

[14] Hayreh SS Prevalent misconceptions about acute retinal vascular occlusive disorders. *Prog. Retin. Eye Res.* 2005;24:493-519.

[15] Rehak J, Rehak M. Branch retinal vein occlusion: pathogenesis, visual prognosis, and treatment modalities. *Curr. Eye Res.* 2008;33:111-31.

[16] Janssen MC, den Heijer M, Cruysberg JR, et al. Retinal vein occlusion: a form of venous thrombosis or a complication of atherosclerosis? A meta-analysis of thrombophilic factors. *Thromb. Haemost.* 2005;93:1021–6.

[17] McIntosh RL, Rogers SL, Lim L, et al. Natural history of central retinal vein occlusion: an evidence-based systematic review. *Ophthalmology* 2010;117:1113-23.

[18] Rogers SL, McIntosh RL, Lim L, et al. Natural history of branch retinal vein occlusion: an evidence-based systematic review. *Ophthalmology* 2010; 117:1094-1101.

[19] D'Amico DJ, Lit ES, Viola F. Lamina puncture for central retinal vein occlusion: results of a pilot trial *Arch. Ophthalmol.* 2006;124:972-7.

[20] Opremcak EM, Bruce RA, Lomeo MD, et al. Radial optic neurotomy for central retinal vein occlusion: a retrospective pilot study of 11 consecutive cases. *Retina* 2001;21:408-15.

[21] Opremcak EM, Rehmar AJ, Ridenour CD, et al. Radial optic neurotomy for central retinal vein occlusion: 117 consecutive cases. *Retina* 2006;26:297-305.

[22] Opremcak EM, Bruce RA. Surgical decompression of branch retinal vein occlusion via arteriovenous crossing sheathotomy: a prospective review of 15 cases. *Retina* 1999;19:1-5.

[23] Weiss JN. Treatment of central retinal vein occlusion by injection of tissue plasminogen activator into a retinal vein *Am. J. Ophthalmol.* 1998;126:142-4.

[24] Weiss JN, Bynoe LA. Injection of tissue plasminogen activator into a branch retinal vein in eyes with central retinal vein occlusion *Ophthalmology* 2001;108;2249-57.

[25] Thach AB, Yau L, Hoang C, et al. Time to clinically significant visual acuity gains after ranibizumab treatment for retinal vein occlusion: BRAVO and CRUISE trials. *Ophthalmology* 2014;121:1059-66.

[26] Laouri M, Chen E, Looman M, et al. The burden of disease of retinal vein occlusion: review of the literature. *Eye* 2011;25:981-8.

[27] Young T, Skatrud J, Peppard PE. Risk factors for obstructive sleep apnea in adults *JAMA* 2004;291:2013-6.

[28] Leroux les Jardins G, Glacet-Bernard A, Lasry S, et al. Retinal vein occlusion and obstructive sleep apnea syndrome [in French]. *J. Fr. Ophthalmol.* 2009;32;420-4.

[29] Tilleul J, Glacet-Bernard A, Coscas G, et al. Underlying conditions associated with the occurrence of retinal vein occlusion [in French]. *J. Fr. Ophthalmol.* 2011;34:318-24.

[30] Yaggi HK, Strohl KP. Adult obstructive sleep apnea /hypopnea syndrome: definitions, risk factors and pathogenesis *Clin. Chest. Med.* 2010;31:179-86.

[31] Gottlieb DJ, Yenokyan G, Newman AB, et al. Prospective study of obstructive sleep apnea and incident coronary heart disease and heart failure: the sleep heart health study. *Circulation* 2010;122:352 60.

[32] Drager LF, Togeiro SM, Polotsy VY, et al. Obstructive sleep apnea: a cardiometabolic risk in obesity and the metabolic syndrome *J. Am. Coll. Cardiol.* 2013;62:569-76.

[33] Kendzerska T, Gershon AS, Hawker G, et al. Obstructive sleep apnea and incident diabetes: a historical cohort study. *Am. J. Respir. Crit. Care* Med 2014;190:218-25.

[34] Guardiola JJ, Matheson PJ, Clavijo LC, et al. Hypercoagulability in patients with obstructive sleep apnea *Sleep Med.* 2001;2:517-23.

[35] Olson LJ, Olson EJ, Somers VK. Obstructive sleep apnea and platelet activation: another potential like between sleep-disordered breathing and cardiovascular disease *Chest* 2004;126:339-41.

[36] Baessler A, Nadeem R, Harvey M, et al. Treatment for sleep apnea by continuous positive airway pressure improves levels of inflammatory markers – a meta-analysis *J. Inflamm.* (Lond) 2013;10:13.

[37] Lui MM, Lam JC, Mak HK, et al. C-reactive protein is associated with obstructive sleep apnea independent of visceral obesity *Chest.* 2009;135:1406.

[38] Namtved SK, Hisdal J, Randby A, et al. Impaired endothelial function in persons with obstructive sleep apnea: impact of obesity *Heart* 2013; 99:30-4.

[39] Govetto A, Dominguez R, Rojas L, et al. Bilateral and simultaneous central retinal vein occlusion in a patient with obstructive sleep apnea syndrome *Case Rep. Ophthalmol.* 2014;5:150-6.

[40] Robinson GV, Pepperell JC, Segal HC, et al. Circulating cardiovascular risk factors in obstructive sleep apnoea: data from randomised controlled trials *Thorax.* 2004;59:777-82.

[41] Leroux les Jardins G, Glacet-Bernard A, Lasry S, et al. Retinal vein occlusion and obstructive sleep apnea syndrome [in French]. *J. Fr. Ophthalmol.* 2009;32;420-4.

In: Eye Diseases …
Editor: Mingwu Wang
ISBN: 978-1-63482-894-9

Chapter 6

Central Serous Chorioretinopathy and Sleep Disorders

Kiersten Pollard, MD, Mingwu Wang, MD, PhD and John Christoforidis*, MD
Department of Ophthalmology and Vision Science,
University of Arizona College of Medicine, AZ, US

Case Presentation

A healthy, 34-year-old, African American man presents with complaints of a black spot affecting his left eye's central vision, which appeared acutely, 1 month before presentation. He reports no associated pain, photophobia, diplopia, or flashing lights. Visual acuity is 20/15 in his right eye, $20/20^{-1}$ in his left eye. Ocular examination is significant for a serous retinal detachment in the left eye, measuring about 1 disk diameter, located in the inferotemporal foveal region (Figure 1A). Optical coherence tomography (OCT) displays a corresponding neurosensory retinal detachment (Figure 1B). Intravenous fluorescein angiography reveals an early phase hyperfluorescent spot in the same area, which gradually enlarges centrifugally through the recirculation

* Email: jchristiforidis@eyes.arizona.edu

phase (Figure 2A, B). The diagnosis of central serous chorioretinopathy (CSC) in the left eye is made.

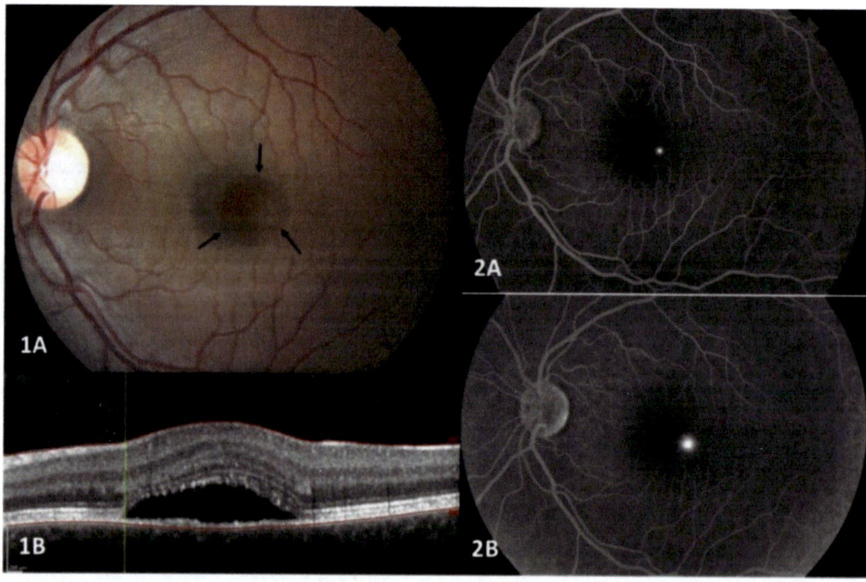

Figure 1. Color fundus photo (1A) showing serous retinal detachment in the left eye, measuring about 1 disk diameter, located in the inferotemporal foveal region. Optical coherence tomography displays a corresponding neurosensory retinal detachment (1B). Intravenous fluorescein angiography (2A, B) reveals an early phase hyperfluorescent spot in the same area, which gradually enlarges centrifugally through the recirculation phase.

The patient denies the use of corticosteroids, in any form, as well as antihistamines He also denied any history of migraines At presentation, he works as a clinical engineer for artificial hearts about 40 hours per week, although the hours are unpredictable, depending on when heart transplant surgeries take place. Seven years previously, he had started training in mixed martial arts and participating in cage fights His daily workout routine is rigorous, often physically quite demanding. In addition, he teaches self-defense classes weekly. He is 6'0" tall with a body mass index of 22.6. His medications include omega-3 fatty acid supplements, glucosamine, as well as modafinil (Provigil, Cephalon, Inc., Frazer, PA) 200 mg by mouth twice daily, for narcolepsy He denied any tobacco, alcohol, or illicit drug use Since other causes of CSC are ruled out, his narcolepsy is believed to be the contributing factor for his CSC and his medications are adjusted. On follow-up after 2 weeks of treatment, his left eye CSC is completely resolved on fundus examination and by OCT.

Central Serous Chorioretinopathy: An Overview

Central serous chorioretinopathy (CSC), also known as central serous rentinopathy, is a common cause of mild to moderate reduced visual acuity. [1] CSC is caused by fluid accumulation from the choroid into the subretinal space, under the retinal pigment epithelium (RPE) or both which leads to symptoms of metamorphopsia, decreased vision, central scotoma and/or micropsia. The “type A” personality and states of duress have long been anecdotally and clinically associated with development of CSC. Recently, more objective evidence from scientific study of the pathophysiology and systemic associations with CSC has identified a link between physiologic stress responses, such as those found in sleep disruptive disorders, and the development of CSC.

Multiple population studies have found that CSC is 2 to 6 times more prevalent in men than in women; [2, 3] and has been associated with states of physiological and psychological stress Much like Takotsubo's Cardiomyopathy, CSC seems to be related to increased sympathomimetic activity during periods of high stress It has been historically and anecdotally described as a disease of the “type A” personality and a disease more likely to be found in those with stressful occupations or personal lives. Several studies report an increased incidence during social turmoil, economic depression. [4] and during times of personal duress. [5] An increased incidence of CSC in patients taking glucocorticoids and those with Cushing's disease has also been reported. [6, 7] Serum cortisol levels are elevated in the late second and third trimester of pregnancy, [8] and pregnancy is also a known risk factor for developing CSC. [9] Additionally, circulating cortisol and catecholemines in patients with CSC have been shown to be elevated by more than 50% above normal values [7] and these levels have been shown to decrease as patients recover.

Most patients present with the complaint of blurry vision Depending on the sizc and location of the fluid accumulation within the retinal tissue, the visual distortion may range from asymptomatic to severe. Patients experience central/paracentral scotomas or metamorphopsia on Amsler grid viewing.

Visual acuity is usually improved with pinhole or plus lenses. Generally CSC affects only one eye at a time but cases of bilateral CSC can also occur. On retinal exam round serous retinal detachment or pigment epithelium detachment can be seen (Figure 1A). RPE atrophy may be noted from prior episodes of CSC in some patients. Active leakage of fluid from the choroid is suggested by subretinal fibrin. [6] Exam findings that have been associated with poor visual outcomes over a 9 year follow up period in one retrospective study included: persistent pigment epithelial detachment and/or subretinal fluid, recurrences, and submacular choroidal neovascularization. [10]

The choroid is one of the most highly vascularized tissues in the body and supplies oxygen and nutrients to the outer retina. [11] The choroid also drains approximately 35% of the aqueous humor from the anterior chamber of the human eye. [12] Unlike retinal vessels, choroidal vessels are fenestrated to allow the passage of low molecular weight molecules, such as glucose and fatty acids, to feed the highly metabolically active photoreceptors. [13] The RPE is a monolayer cellular membrane that sits between the choroid and the photoreceptors, and functions as part of the retinal-blood barrier. [14] Light energy focused by the lens of the eye onto the retina is also absorbed by the pigmented cells in the RPE reducing photo-oxidative damage and light scatter. [15] The nutrients from the choroid are preferentially pumped across the RPE to feed the photoreceptors, and metabolic waste products that accumulate in the sub-retinal space are transported back across the RPE to the choroid for elimination. Due to the delicate balance established by these two structures, dysfunction of either the choroid or the RPE has immediate detrimental effects on vision

The pathophysiology of CSC is not entirely understood, but with advances in ocular imaging more of the development and potential causes of this disease are becoming clearer. In CSC the choroidal vessels appear to become hyperpermeable as noted on indocyanine green angiography. [16] This is hypothesized to occur secondary to the usual culprits that cause changes in osmotic or pressure gradients leading to increased vascular permeability: toxins, stasis or inflammation (infectious or immunological). The association of CSC with states of increased glucocorticoids and catecholamines would suggest that these chemicals affect choroidal permeability or RPE barrier function.

Corticosteroids have been shown to potentiate vasoactive response to norepinephrine in vascular studies. [17] Further evidence that catecholamines and glucocorticoids may affect choroid permeability is presented in a 1982 monkey model of CSC. [18] This model showed that after serial injections of norepinephrine alone, or after serial injections of norepinephrine and prednisolone, pigment epithelium detachments occurred in the eyes of the 2 monkeys studied. Additionally the fluorescein angiographic findings were similar to those found in human CSC. This animal study described damage to choriocapillaries and the RPE leading to fluid leakage from the choroid with associated RPE detachments. A proposed mechanism of action for the involvement of the RPE in CSC is that as hydrostatic pressure increases, from choroidal hyperpearmeability, the barrier function of the RPE breaks down and fluid accumulates below the retina. [19] This would lead to the RPE detachments noted on exam and the fluid leakage seen on fluorescein angiography (Figure 2A, B).

CSC may be acute or chronic in time course, a singular event or a recurring problem. The clinical definition of chronic CSC is the presence of subretinal fluid for greater than 3 months. While acute CSC is the most common form and generally resolves on its own with no permanent visual loss, chronic, or recurrent CSC can lead to photoreceptor death, and central neovascularization The vast majority of patients who develop acute CSC do not go on to develop chronic, or recurrent CSC, and to date there is little understanding of the risk factors that predispose a patient to developing chronic CSC. This lack of initial prediction of severity makes regular follow up and communication of possible clinical outcomes to patients especially important. Foveal photoreceptor atrophy has been noted to occur after 4 months of symptoms in patients with CSC. [20] Atrophic changes of the foveal photoreceptors may lead to permanent visual loss and therefore it has been recommended that patients with symptomatic CSC for greater than 3 consecutive months undergo treatment to prevent permanent atrophy. [21] The first line of treatment in patients taking systemic glucocorticoids is to reduce the total dose of glucocorticoids, as this has been shown to lead to resolution of CSC. Patients with endogenous hypercortisolism should receive appropriate treatment for the underlying cause. In the case of life threatening disease processes requiring high dose systemic steroids and the development of CSC, eye physicians and internists should work together with the patient to optimize systemic disease outcomes and preserve sight in accordance with the patient's individual quality of life goals.

In patients without endogenous or external hypercortisolism there are currently several options for treatment Photodynamic therapy is the mainstay of treatment for chronic CSC as it has been shown to improve visual acuity. [22] Photodynamic therapy likely works by sealing leaky choriocapillaries resulting in reduced permeability and reduced exudative fluid. [23] While photodynamic therapy is effective it is not without side effects, which include: RPE tears, neovascularization and ischemia. [24] These side effects are reduced with the use of half dose or half fluence treatment. [25] Other treatments are still under investigation as none seem to effect long term visual acuity in randomized controlled trials Argon laser photocoagulation has been shown to reduce initial rehabilitation time, but in the long term has not been shown to affect final visual acuity or reduce recurrence rates of CSC. [26] Intravitreal bevacizumab is currently being studied as a treatment for chronic CSC and appears to reduce subretinal fluid in these cases. [27, 28] Studies of the long term effect of this treatment may have on visual acuity have not been completed at this time.

Sleep Apnea and Central Serous Chorioretinopathy

An increasing number of diseases are being associated with obstructive sleep apnea (OSA) as more is learned about its pathophysiology and its effects on the body. Several recent studies have found the prevalence of OSA among patients with CSC to be significantly higher than in the general population. [29, 30] The link between these two seemingly disparate diseases is made clearer when the pathophysiology of OSA is understood. OSA is a cyclic process in which the patient's upper airway constricts, causing asphyxia This asphyxia causes autonomic arousal such that the patient can gain control of their airway and resolve the hypoxia When the autonomic arousal is diminished (when the patient falls back to sleep), the airway constricts and the whole process begins again. A group of British physicians astutely described this in 1870 as "fruitless contractions of the inspiratory and expiratory muscles against glottic obstruction with accompanying cyanosis during sleep." [31] This cycle of "fruitless contractions" results in many episodes of nocturnal awakenings preventing the patient from getting the continuous sleep needed to feel rested the next day. The signs and symptoms of OSA were described by Dickens years prior to the British medical community's published notice of the disease. His character, Fat Boy Joe, in *The Pickwick Papers* [32] was noted to be

> "a wonderfully fat boy–habited as a serving lad, standing upright on the mat, with his eyes closed as if in sleep [...] "Sleep!" said the old gentleman, 'he's always asleep. Goes on errands fast asleep, and snores as he waits at table."

The effects of OSA extend far beyond daytime somnolence, however, as patients are greater than 2 times more likely to die of cardiovascular events than people without OSA, [33] are two times more likely to be involved in motor vehicle accidents [34] and most of whom develop hypertension increasing their risk for heart and renal failure There are several exam findings which suggest OSA may be present, including: small recessed jaw, obesity – especially in patients with large amounts of adipose tissue in the neck, elevated blood pressure, and daytime somnolence.

As noted previously, CSC has been associated with abnormally high serum levels of glucocorticoids and catecholamines Cyclic awakenings and abnormal sleep patterns, like those in OSA and narcolepsy, are associated with pulsatile cortisol release. [35] Patients with untreated OSA have been found to have increased circulating catecholamines [36] and the amount of catecholamines has been found to correlate to the severity of apnea. [37] Recently a survey of CSC patients and control subjects matched, not just for age and gender, but also for body mass index found no statistical difference between the incidences of OSA between groups. [38] This study used the Berlin Questionnaire [39] to classify patients as "high risk" for OSA and grouped people at "high risk" with those who were diagnosed with OSA by sleep study. As not all people who are "high risk" truly have OSA it is difficult to interpret these recent findings and more research is ongoing.

Given the increased morbidity and mortality of untreated OSA, optometrists and ophthalmologists should screen CSC patients during history-taking for signs and symptoms of OSA and refer appropriate patients for further work up. An appropriate initial screening test is the Epworth Sleep Scale [40] which patients can fill out on their own and present to their primary care doctor or sleep specialist for review.

The initial and most effective therapy for OSA is continuous positive airway pressure (CPAP) which prevents the collapse of the airway during sleep, eliminating the episodes of hypoxic apnea and pulsatile cortisol release. Long term CPAP treatment has been shown to decrease the overall norepinephrine to levels found in non-apneic individuals. [41] There are case reports of the rapid resolution of CSC in OSA patients who began CPAP without ophthalmologic intervention, [42] further strengthening the link between OSA and the development of CSC.

There have been case reports of other disorders which cause disruptions in sleep patterns and the development of recurrent CSC, such as narcolepsy. [43] Treatment of this underlying sleep disruptive disease was also shown to lead to the resolution of CSC.

OSA is a modifiable risk factor for the development of many diseases, including CSC. Treatment of OSA can prevent patients from developing recurring or chronic CSC. This is important because the current interventional ophthalmologic therapies have been primarily temporizing, often followed by recurrences of CSC and without significant improvement on long term visual acuity outcomes. The correlation between OSA and CSC is not well-recognized, yet its awareness by both the treating primary care physicians and eye physicians may serve to improve the visual outcomes and the general health of these patients.

References

[1] Wang M, Munch IC, Hasler PW, Prunte C, et al. Central Serous Retinopathy. *Acta. Ophthalmologica* 2008; 86:126-145.

[2] Liew G, Quin G, Gillies M, Fraser-Bell S. Central Serous Chorioretinopathy: A Review of Epidemiology and Pathophysiology. *Clin. Experiment Ophthalmol.* 2013;41:201-14.

[3] Tsai DC, Chen SJ, Huang CC, et al. Epidemiology of Idiopathic Central Serous Chorioretinopathy in Taiwan, 2001-2006: A Population-Based Study. *PLoS One* 2013 Jun 24;8(6):e66858.

[4] Rouvas AA, Chatziralli IP, Ladas ID, et al. The Impact of Financial Crisis on Central Serous Chorioretinopathy in Greece: Is There Any Correlation? *Eur. J. Ophthalmol.* 2014;24:559-65.

[5] Conrad R, Bodeewes I, Schilling G, et al. Central Serous Chorioretinopathy and Psychological Stress. *Ophthalmologe* 2000;97:527-31.

[6] Friedman N, Kaiser P, Pineda R, eds The Massachusetts Eye and Ear Infirmary Illustrated Manual of Ophthamology. [Kindle Edition.] 3rd ed. Elservier Saunders; 2009:8617-64.

[7] Garg SP, Dada T, Talwar D, Biswas NR. Endogenous Cortisol Profile in Patients with Central Serous Chorioretinopathy. *Br. J. Ophthalmol.* 1997; 81:962-4.

[8] Cousins L, Rigg L, Hollingsworth D, et al. Qualitative and Quantitative Assessment of the Circadian Rhythm of Cortisol in Pregnancy. *Am. J.* Obstet Gynecol 1983; 145:411-6.

[9] Haimovici R, Koh S, Gagnon DR, et al. Risk Factors for Central Serous Chorioretinopathy: A Case-Control Study. *Ophthalmology* 2004; 111:244-9.

[10] Loo RH, Scott IU, Flynn H Jr, et al. Factors Associated With Reduced Visual Acuity During Long-Term Follow-Up of Patients with Idiopathic Central Serous Chorioretinopathy. *Retina* 2002; 22:19-24.

[11] Nickla DL, Wallman J. The Multifunctional Choroid. *Prog. Retin. Eye* Res 2010;29:144-68.

[12] Alm A, Nilsson SF. Uveoscleral Outflow: *A Review. Exp. Eye Res.* 2009;88:760-8.

[13] Bill A, Törnquist P, Alm A. Permeability of the Intraocular Blood Vessels. *Trans. Ophthalmol. Soc.* UK 1980;100:332-6.

[14] Bok D. The Retinal Pigment Epithelium: A Versatile Partner in Vision. *J. Cell Sci. Suppl.* 1993;17: 189–195.

[15] Boulton M, Dayhaw-Barker P. The Role of the Retinal Pigment Epithelium: Topographical Variation and Ageing Changes. *Eye* 2001;15:384–9.

[16] Okushiba U, Takeda M. Study of Choroidal Vascular Lesions in Central Serous Chorioretinopathy Using Indocyanine Green Angiography [In Japanese]. *Nihon Ganka Gakkai Zasshi* 1997;101:74-82.

[17] Yang S, Zhang L. Glucocorticoids and Vascular Reactivity. *Curr. Vasc. Pharmacol.* 2004;2:1-12.

[18] Yoshioka H, Katsume Y, Akune H. Experimental Central Serous Chorioretinopathy in Monkey Eyes: Fluorescein Angiographic Findings. *Ophthalmologica* 1982;185:168-78.

[19] Nicholson B, Noble J, Forooghian F, et al. Central Serous Chorioretinopathy: Update on Pathophysiology and Treatment. *Surv. Ophthalmol.* 2013;58:103-26.

[20] Wang MS, Sander B, Larsen M. Retinal Atrophy in Idiopathic Central Serous Chorioretinopathy. *Am. J. Ophthalmol.* 2002;133:787-93.

[21] Gemenetzil M, De Salvo G, Lotery AJ. Central Serous Chorioretinopathy: An Update on Pathogenesis and Treatment. *Eye* 2010;24:1743–56.

[22] Taban M, Boyer DS, Thomas EL, Taban M. Chronic Central Serous Chorioretinopathy: Photodynamic Therapy. *Am. J. Ophthalmol* 2004;137:1073-80.

[23] Chan WM, Lam DS, Lai TY, et al. Choroidal Vascular Remodelling in Central Serous Chorioretinopathy after Indocyanine Green Guided Photodynamic Therapy with Verteporfin: A Novel Treatment at the Primary Disease Level. *Br. J. Ophthalmol.* 2003;87:1453-8.

[24] Lee PY, Kim KS, Lee WK. Severe Choroidal Ischemia Following Photodynamic Therapy for Pigment Epithelial Detachment and Chronic Central Serous Chorioretinopathy. *Jpn. J. Ophthalmol.* 2009; 53:52-6.

[25] Rouvas A, Stavrakas P, Theodossiadis PG, et al. Long-Term Results of Half-Fluence Photodynamic Therapy for Chronic Central Serous Chorioretinopathy. *Eur. J. Ophthalmol.* 2012;22:417-22.

[26] Ficker L, Vafidis G, While A, Leaver P. Long-Term Follow-Up of a Prospective Trial of Argon Laser Photocoagulation in the Treatment of Central Serous Retinopathy. *Br. J. Ophthalmol.* 1988;72:829-34.

[27] Schaal KB, Hoeh AE, Scheuerle A, et al. Intravitreal Bevacizumab for Treatment of Chronic Central Serous Chorioretinopathy. European *Journal of Ophthalmology* 2009;19:613-7.

[28] Artunay O, Yuzbasioglu E, Rasier, et al. Intravitreal Bevacizumab in Treatment of Idiopathic Persistent Central Serous Chorioretinopathy: A Prospective, Controlled Clinical Study. *Current Eye Research* 2010;35:91-8.

[29] Leveque TK, Yu L, Musch DC, et al. Central Serous Chorioretinopathy and Risk for Obstructive Sleep Apnea. *Sleep Breath* 2007;11:253-7.

[30] Kloos P, Laube I, Thoelen A. Obstructive Sleep Apnea in Patients with Central Serous Chorioretinopathy. *Graefes Arch. Clin. Exp. Ophthalmol.* 2008;246:1225-8.

[31] Lavie P. Restless Nights: Understanding Snoring and Sleep Apnea. New Haven, CT: Yale Univ. Press, 2003.

[32] Dickens, C. The Posthumous Papers of the Pickwick Club. London; New York. Penguin Books, 1999.

[33] Fonseca MI, Pereira T, Caseiro P. Death and Disability in Patients with Sleep Apnea - A Meta-analysis [in Portugese]. *Arq. Bras. Cardiol.* 2015;104:58-66.

[34] Basoglu OK, Tasbakan MS. Elevated Risk of Sleepiness-Related Motor Vehicle Accidents in Patients with Obstructive Sleep Apnea Syndrome: A Case-Control Study. *Traffic Inj. Prev.* 2014;15:470-6.

[35] Spath-Schwalbe E, Gofferje M, Kern W, Born J, et al. Sleep Disruption Alters Nocturnal ACTH and Cortisol Secretory Patterns. *Biol. Psychiatry* 1999;29:575 84.

[36] Fletcher EC, Miller J, Schaaf JW, Fletcher JG. Urinary Catecholamines Before and After Tracheostomy in Patients with Obstructive Sleep Apnea and Hypertension. *Sleep* 1987;10:35-44.

[37] Eisenberg E, Zimlichman R, Lavie P. Plasma Norepinephrine Levels in Patients with Sleep Apnea Syndrome. *New Eng. J. of Med.* 1990;322:932-3.

[38] Brodie FL, Charlson ES, Aleman TS, et al. Obstructive Sleep Apnea and Central Serous Chorioretinopathy. *Retina* 2015 Feb;35(2):238-43.

[39] Netzer NC, Stoohs RA, Netzer CM, et al. Using the Berlin Questionnaire to Identify Patients at Risk for the Sleep Apnea Syndrome. *Ann. Intern. Med.* 1999;131:485-91.

[40] Johns MW. A New Method for Measuring Daytime Sleepiness: The Epworth Sleepiness Scale. *Sleep* 1991;14:540-5.

[41] Hedner J, Darpo B, Ejnell H, J et al. Reduction in Sympathetic Activity after Long-Term CPAP Treatment in Sleep Apnoea: Cardiovascular Implications. *European Respiratory Journal 1995;8:222-229.*

[42] Jain AK, Kaines A, Schwartz S. Bilateral Central Serous Chorioretinopathy Resolving Rapidly with Treatment for Obstructive Sleep Apnea. *Graefes Arch. Clin. Exp. Ophthalmol.* 2010;248:1037-9.

[43] Kim JT, Eichling PS, Wang M. Central Serous Chorioretinopathy Associated with Narcolepsy. *Retin. Cases Brief Rep.* 2011;5:302-5.

In: Eye Diseases …
Editor: Mingwu Wang
ISBN: 978-1-63482-894-9

Chapter 7

Diabetic Retinopathy and Obstructive Sleep Apnea

***Samuel C. Werner, MD and John Christoforidis**[*], MD*
Department of Ophthalmology and Vision Science,
University of Arizona College of Medicine, AZ, US

Case Presentation

A 45-year old woman with morbid obesity and a 19-year history of type 1 diabetes mellitus presents with a complaint of blurring vision of the left eye that occurred gradually and painlessly over the past 6 months. Best-corrected vision is 20/200 in the affected eye. Dilated funduscopic examination reveals evidence of macular edema, hard exudates, and neovascularization Fluorescein angiography is performed which confirms widespread retinal ischemia and macular vasculature leakage A diagnosis of proliferative diabetic retinopathy with clinically significant macular edema is made.

[*] Corresponding author: jchristoforidis@eyes.arizona.edu.

Diabetic Retinopathy: An Overview

Diabetic retinopathy (DR) is one of the leading causes of blindness worldwide While early disease is usually asymptomatic, more severe cases can result in retinal ischemia and neovascularization, intraretinal and vitreous hemorrhages, neovascular glaucoma, preretinal fibrosis and traction retinal detachment, causing potentially irreversible vision loss. It is now the most common etiology for newly diagnosed blindness in adults aged 25-74.[1] In 2012, it was estimated that 93 million people suffer from DR worldwide, or roughly one third of all diabetics. Of these, a projected 21 million suffer from a severe form of retinopathy that is visually threatening and this number is estimated to increase dramatically by 2030. [2, 3] DR is considered a heterogeneous disorder with many clinical etiologies linked to the development of the disease, including obstructive sleep apnea (OSA).

The natural history of DR has been well-characterized as a highly specific vascular condition of type 1 and type 2 diabetes The disease process occurs as a result of increased permeability in retinal vasculature causing ischemia and new blood vessel growth Loss of retinal microvascular cells, specifically pericytes and endothelial cells, has been shown to occur early in the disease. [4] As these cells are lost, microaneurysms in retinal vasculature begin to occur. These focal dilations (Figure 1) are usually the earliest signs of DR and are found in most diabetics who have had the disease for more than 20 years. [5] With increasing vascular permeability, fluid begins to leak into the retina As this fluid is resorbed, hard exudates composed of lipid and proteinaceous material are left behind (Figure 2). This leakage results in macular edema which can have significant impact on vision if it occurs near the macula (Figure 3). In several large studies, incidence of macular edema over a ten-year period was found to be roughly one in five for insulin-dependent diabetic patients. [6] As the disease progresses, vasculature becomes further compromised leading to ischemic retinopathy with ensuing neovascularization Fragile new vessels can rupture resulting in vitreous hemorrhage (Figure 4). New blood vessels can also generate fibrous overgrowths that may distort the underlying retina or trigger tractional forms of retinal detachment (Figure 5). Significant neovascularization, if left untreated, carries a 60% risk of severe vision loss in 5 years. [7] Pathogenesis of DR is complex and not completely understood. Investigation into cellular metabolism, signaling, and inflammation has revealed a variety of risk factors associated with the development of the disease including a possible connection to OSA. This connection, along with what is currently known regarding the pathogenesis of DR will be discussed in the latter half of this chapter.

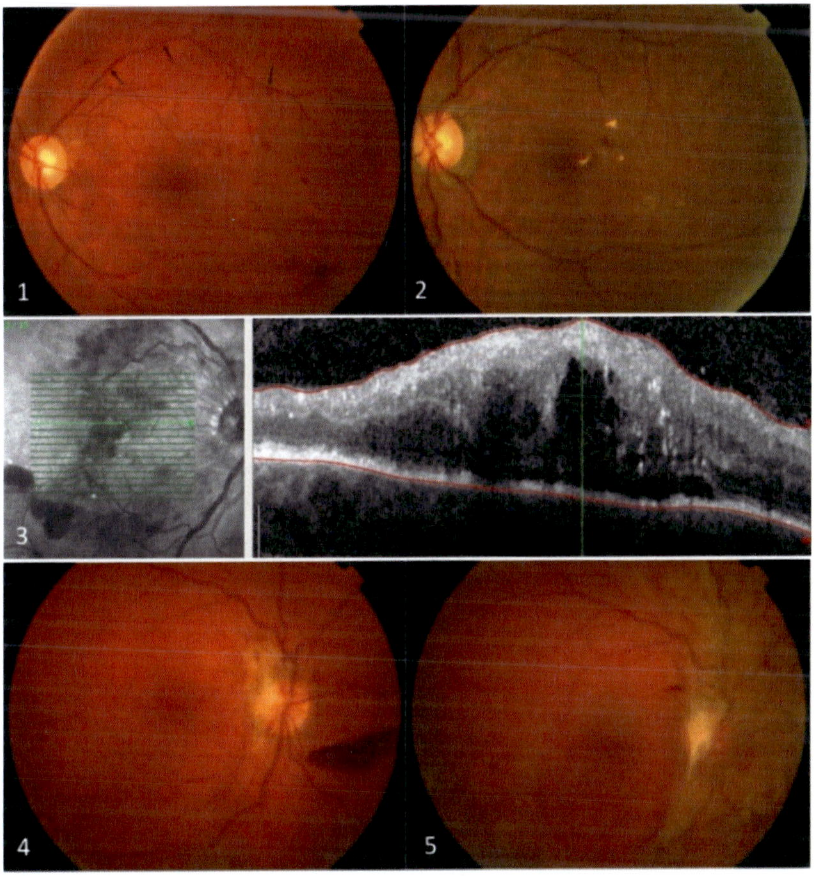

Figure 1. Focal dilitations (arrows) in a patient with non-proliferative diabetic retinopathy. Figure 2. Fundus photography demonstrating non-proliferative diabetic retinopathy with the presence of exudates, dot-blot hemorrhages and microaneurysms. Figure 3. Spectral domain optical coherence tomography with Heidelberg Spectralis® demonstrating profound diabetic macular edema in a patient with proliferative diabetic retinopathy. Figure 4. Color fundus photograph in a patient with proliferative diabetic retinopathy demonstrating the presence of a 'boat shaped' preretinal and subhyaloidal hemorrhage nasal to the optic nerve and inferior to neovascular vessels, preretinal fibrosis overlying the optic nerve and the proximal portions of the temporal vascular arcades and dot-blot hemorrhages mostly in the temporal portion of the macula. Figure 5. Color fundus photograph demonstrating the presence of dense preretinal proliferative fibrous tissue overlying the optic nerve and the vascular temporal arcades. This patient is at high risk for developing a traction retinal detachment.

Development of DR is considered a multifactorial process that is influenced by a variety of risk factors Large epidemiologic studies involving over 10,000 diabetic patients in the 1980s revealed a strong correlation between the duration of diabetes and the occurrence of DR, with prevalence varying from 28.8% in patients with diabetes for less than five years compared to 77.8% in those having diabetes for more than 15 years. [8] Other factors shown to increase the risk of developing retinopathy were poor glycemic control, nephropathy, and hypertension. [9-11] Independent of these known risk factors, DR is more common in African-Americans and Hispanics. [12,13] The majority of populations examined show a correlation between obesity and DR, [14-16] though conflicting findings have been published including a recent study demonstrating a lower prevalence of retinopathy in obese diabetics. [17, 18, 19] This discrepancy in findings may be related to variations in study populations, but the influence of obesity as a risk factor for retinopathy is not yet defined. [16] Significant research efforts have been made to determine genetic factors associated with DR. Familial and twin studies have demonstrated a clear hereditary tendency to the development of DR. [20-24] A large diabetes complications trial found a three-fold increase of severe DR in relatives of patients with retinopathy compared to patients with no signs of ocular diabetic complications. [25] These familial aggregation studies suggest genetic influences affect the prevalence and severity of DR. [24] Despite this, the search for specific genetic links has yielded only weak associations that have not been replicated. [24, 26, 27] No genes are currently identified as high risk for developing DR. [27] Genome wide association studies and linkage analyses have however pointed towards novel pathways in glucose metabolism, inflammation, and angiogenesis, leading investigators to consider a variety of new risk factors and potential treatment options.

Management of DR depends largely on classification and severity. Two classifications exist for the disease, nonproliferative diabetic retinopathy (NPDR) and proliferative diabetic retinopathy (PDR). PDR is characterized by the presence of pathologic new vasculature in the retina, whereas NPDR lacks this neovasculature. Both can be further characterized by severity to predict risk of progression and determine appropriate treatment. [28] Mild to moderate NPDR is typically asymptomatic and managed with regular screening for progression. [29] More severe cases may require laser panretinal photocoagulation to reduce the risk of developing PDR. [30, 31] For patients with PDR, panretinal photocoagulation has been shown to slow progression and significantly reduce the risk of severe vision loss. [32] Adjunct therapies can include vascular endothelial growth factor (VEGF) inhibitors to reduce neovascularization and vitrectomy to clear vitreous hemorrhage. [33, 34] Macular edema, which can occur at any stage of DR, is typically treated with intravitreal VEGF inhibitors and focal laser photocoagulation. [35, 36] Surgical removal of the vitreous, posterior hyaloid and internal limiting membrane is sometimes performed for cases that are refractive to medical and laser therapies. [37] Because disease progression can be rapid, regular screening for DR is a critical component of effective treatment. [5, 38]

Diabetic Retinopathy and the Link to Obstructive Sleep Apnea

OSA is a widely prevalent and under-diagnosed breathing disorder. [39] An estimated 15% of the US population suffers from OSA, a number that increases to 23% and 86% in diabetic and obese diabetic populations, respectively. [39-41] Hypoxic episodes from untreated OSA are known to cause systemic sympathetic surges and inflammation associated with worsening insulin resistance, atherosclerosis, hypertension, and cardiovascular mortality risk. [42-44] Increasing evidence suggests a connection between OSA and DR. Numerous studies have examined the prevalence of OSA in patients with DR. These studies have predominantly determined OSA to be strongly associated with presence of DR, independent of known risk factors for retinopathy. [45, 46, 51, 52] Retinopathy scores used to evaluate disease are noted to be much poorer in groups diagnosed with OSA and complications involving the macula occur 3 times more frequently in subjects with OSA. [44, 45] In one observational study, over half of individuals with diabetic macular edema who underwent sleep studies showed evidence of OSA. [47] There is also evidence that OSA may worsen the progression of retinopathy.[48] Roughly half of subjects with sight-threatening DR were found to have OSA compared to only 29% of those with non-sight-threatening retinopathy. [48] Greater nocturnal oxygen desaturations are also noted in individuals with more advanced retinopathy, suggesting the severity of OSA correlates with severity of DR. [49] Association between OSA and DR persists even after adjustment for conventional and novel biomarkers for retinopathy, establishing OSA as a potentially important independent predictor of retinopathy. [50]

The mechanism by which OSA and DR are connected is presently unknown. Recurrent episodes of intermittent hypoxia, sympathetic catecholamine release, re-oxygenation, and blood pressure spikes have all been proposed as possible means by which OSA affects the retina However, the complex pathogenesis of DR is not completely understood and the effects of OSA on disease progression even less so. [45, 48, 53] Development of microvascular diabetic complications has been strongly linked to the effects of hyperglycemia and several extensively described intracellular pathways including the formation of advanced glycation end products, protein kinase C activation, and increased polyol/hexosamine pathway flux. [53-56] Disruption of these cellular functions occurs via a single unifying mechanism of increased oxidative stress, [57, 58] and it is through additional hypoxia and oxidative stress that OSA is proposed to influence DR. [59] Evidence of this comes from studies showing increased levels of inflammatory biomarkers associated with oxidative stress and DR in patients with OSA. [60, 61] Levels of VEGF are elevated with OSA, a growth factor triggered by oxidative stress and strongly linked to the development of DR. [60] These increased levels of inflammatory growth factors may influence retinopathy treatment outcomes. [62] Patients with poor response to anti-VEGF therapy for DR were shown to have a higher prevalence of OSA. [62]

The retina has the highest oxygen uptake of any tissue, making it exceptionally sensitive to hypoxia and oxidative stress. [63] Analysis of oxygen tension within retina tissue shows available oxygen to be near zero when energy demand is high, suggesting that normally functioning retinal cells are on the verge of hypoxia and their capacity to compensate for disease is limited. [64, 65] Indeed, in diabetic patients with no signs of DR, deficits can be measured in color vision, contrast sensitivity, and electrophysiological response. [66, 67] These deficits are quickly reversed by oxygen inhalation suggesting the diabetic retina suffers from hypoxia early in the disease. [68] Additionally, diabetics with coexisting diseases that damage photoreceptors in the retina, thereby reducing oxygen demand of the retina, rarely develop signs of DR, despite exhibiting advanced diabetic vascular complications in other organs. [69, 70] Oxygen demands of the retina are highest in the dark, or during sleep, and it is during this vulnerable period that short intervals of hypoxia brought about by OSA can exacerbate DR. [59] Taken together, this evidence suggests hypoxia, brought about by high tissue metabolic demand and limited oxygen availability, is central in the pathogenesis of DR and a likely mechanism for the association with OSA.

Efforts to treat DR by reducing retinal hypoxia either by reducing oxygen demand or treating OSA have yielded interesting results. Administering supplemental nasal oxygen to patients with DR was found to cause reduction in diabetic macular edema. [71] Because retinal oxygen demand increases by as much as two-fold in the dark, rather than providing supplemental oxygen, one small study and a phase II trial have investigated the effects of preventing dark adaptation on DR. [72, 73] Exposing patients with DR to minimal amounts of illumination through closed eyelids at night significantly reduced progression and even reversed signs of retinopathy. [72, 73] A phase III trial is currently underway to better establish the efficacy of this treatment, but these promising early results again implicate retinal hypoxia in the development of DR and the relationship to OSA. Standard treatment of OSA utilizes mild air pressure in the form of continuous positive airway pressure (CPAP) to maintain an open airway and prevent apneic and hypoxic events. As of now, no large trials have explored the effect of treating OSA on DR. A small study investigating CPAP use in subjects with DR and OSA found that patients with high CPAP compliance had one line visual improvement over a period of six months compared to CPAP users with low-compliance. [74] These initial favorable results hint at potential benefits to preventing hypoxic episodes at night when the retina is susceptible to oxidative stress Additional prospective and interventional studies are needed establish the impact of treating OSA on the progression of DR.

Accumulating evidence suggests a convincing connection between OSA and DR. Although the exact mechanism relating these diseases has yet to be defined, literature supports the model of increased oxidative stress imposed by OSA on retina tissue in diabetic patients While treating OSA provides a clear benefit to cardiovascular morbidity and mortality, it remains to be seen whether management of OSA improves outcomes for DR. Even so, multifactorial risk reduction strategies remain essential to the prevention of diabetic complications and healthcare professionals in primary care, sleep medicine, and ophthalmology should be aware of the link between OSA and DR.

References

[1] Standards of medical care in diabetes--2014. *Diabetes Care*, 2014, 37 Suppl 1, S14-80.

[2] Yau, JW; Rogers, SL; Kawasaki, R; et al. Global prevalence and major risk factors of diabetic retinopathy *Diabetes Care*, 2012, 35(3), 556-64.

[3] Wild, S; Roglic, G; Green, A; Sicree, R; King, H. Global prevalence of diabetes, estimates for the year 2000 and projections for 2030. *Diabetes Care*, 2004, 27(5), 1047-53.

[4] Mizutani, M; Kern, TS; Lorenzi, M. Accelerated death of retinal microvascular cells in human and experimental diabetic retinopathy *J Clin Invest*, 1996, 97(12), 2883-90.

[5] Klein, R; Klein, BE; Moss, SE; Davis, MD; Demets, DL. The Wisconsin epidemiologic study of diabetic retinopathy III. Prevalence and risk of diabetic retinopathy when age at diagnosis is 30 or more years. *Arch Ophthalmol*, 1984, 102(4), 527-32.

[6] Klein, R; Klein, BE; Moss, SE; Cruickshanks, KJ. The Wisconsin Epidemiologic Study of Diabetic Retinopathy. XV. The long-term incidence of macular edema *Ophthalmology*, 1995, 102(1), 7-16.

[7] Fundus photographic risk factors for progression of diabetic retinopathy ETDRS report number 12. Early Treatment Diabetic Retinopathy Study Research Group. *Ophthalmology*, 1991, 98(5 Suppl), 823-33.

[8] Klein, R; Klein, BE; Moss, SE; Davis, MD; Demets, DL. The Wisconsin epidemiologic study of diabetic retinopathy III. Prevalence and risk of diabetic retinopathy when age at diagnosis is 30 or more years. *Arch Ophthalmol*, 1984, 102(4), 527-32.

[9] Klein, R. Hyperglycemia and microvascular and macrovascular disease in diabetes *Diabetes Care*, 1995, 18(2), 258-68.

[10] Estacio, RO; Mcfarling, E; Biggerstaff, S; Jeffers, BW; Johnson, D; Schrier, RW. Overt albuminuria predicts diabetic retinopathy in Hispanics with NIDDM. *Am J Kidney Dis*, 1998, 31(6), 947-53.

[11] Leske, MC; Wu, SY; Hennis, A; et al. Hyperglycemia, blood pressure, and the 9-year incidence of diabetic retinopathy: the Barbados Eye Studies. *Ophthalmology*, 2005, 112(5), 799-805.

[12] Emanuele, N; Sacks, J; Klein, R; et al. Ethnicity, race, and baseline retinopathy correlates in the veterans affairs diabetes trial *Diabetes Care*, 2005, 28(8), 1954-8.

[13] Harris, EL; Sherman, SH; Georgopoulos, A. Black-white differences in risk of developing retinopathy among individuals with type 2 diabetes *Diabetes Care*, 1999, 22(5), 779-83.

[14] Kaštelan, S; Tomić, M; Gverović antunica, A; Ljubić, S; Salopek rabatić, J; Karabatić, M. Body mass index, a risk factor for retinopathy in type 2 diabetic patients *Mediators Inflamm*, 2013, 2013, 436329.

[15] Dirani, M; Xie, J; Fenwick, E; et al. Are obesity and anthropometry risk factors for diabetic retinopathy? The diabetes management project *Invest Ophthalmol Vis Sci*, 2011, 52(7), 4416-21.

[16] Song, SJ; Wong, TY. Current concepts in diabetic retinopathy *Diabetes Metab J*, 2014, 38(6), 416-25.

[17] Klein, R; Klein, BE; Moss, SE. Is obesity related to microvascular and macrovascular complications in diabetes? The Wisconsin Epidemiologic Study of Diabetic Retinopathy. *Arch Intern Med*, 1997, 157(6), 650-6.

[18] Rooney, D; Lye, WK; Tan, G; et al. Body mass index and retinopathy in Asian populations with diabetes mellitus *Acta Diabetol*, 2014,

[19] Lu, J; Hou, X; Zhang, L; et al. Association between body mass index and diabetic retinopathy in Chinese patients with type 2 diabetes *Acta Diabetol*, 2015.

[20] Leslie, RD; Pyke, DA. Diabetic retinopathy in identical twins *Diabetes*, 1982, 31(1), 19-21.

[21] Clustering of long-term complications in families with diabetes in the diabetes control and complications trial The Diabetes Control and Complications Trial Research Group. *Diabetes*, 1997, 46(11), 1829-39.

[22] Hietala K; Forsblom C; Summanen P; Groop PH. Heritability of proliferative diabetic retinopathy *Diabetes*, 2008, 57(8), 2176-80.

[23] Rema, M; Saravanan, G; Deepa, R; Mohan, V. Familial clustering of diabetic retinopathy in South Indian Type 2 diabetic patients *Diabet Med*, 2002, 19(11), 910-6.

[24] Liew, G; Klein, R; Wong, TY. The role of genetics in susceptibility to diabetic retinopathy *Int Ophthalmol Clin*, 2009, 49(2), 35-52.

[25] Clustering of long-term complications in families with diabetes in the diabetes control and complications trial The Diabetes Control and Complications Trial Research Group. *Diabetes*, 1997, 46(11), 1829-39.

[26] Ng, DP. Human genetics of diabetic retinopathy: current perspectives. *J Ophthalmol*, 2010, 2010

[27] Kuo, JZ; Wong, TY; Rotter, JI. Challenges in elucidating the genetics of diabetic retinopathy *JAMA Ophthalmol*, 2014, 132(1), 96-107.

[28] Aiello, LM. Perspectives on diabetic retinopathy *Am J Ophthalmol*, 2003, 136(1), 122-35.

[29] Younis, N; Broadbent, DM; Vora, JP; Harding, SP Incidence of sight-threatening retinopathy in patients with type 2 diabetes in the Liverpool Diabetic Eye Study, a cohort study. *Lancet*, 2003, 361(9353), 195-200.

[30] Lövestam-adrian, M; Agardh, CD; Torffvit, O; Agardh, E. Type 1 diabetes patients with severe non-proliferative retinopathy may benefit

from panretinal photocoagulation *Acta Ophthalmol Scand*, 2003, 81(3), 221-5.

[31] Early photocoagulation for diabetic retinopathy ETDRS report number 9. Early Treatment Diabetic Retinopathy Study Research Group. *Ophthalmology*, 1991, 98(5 Suppl), 766-85.

[32] Photocoagulation treatment of proliferative diabetic retinopathy Clinical application of Diabetic Retinopathy Study (DRS) findings, DRS Report Number 8. The Diabetic Retinopathy Study Research Group. *Ophthalmology*, 1981, 88(7), 583-600.

[33] Googe, J; Brucker, AJ; Bressler, NM; et al. Randomized trial evaluating short-term effects of intravitreal ranibizumab or triamcinolone acetonide on macular edema after focal/grid laser for diabetic macular edema in eyes also receiving panretinal photocoagulation Retina (Philadelphia, Pa) 2011, 31(6), 1009-27.

[34] Early vitrectomy for severe vitreous hemorrhage in diabetic retinopathy Four-year results of a randomized trial: Diabetic Retinopathy Vitrectomy Study Report 5. *Arch Ophthalmol*, 1990, 108(7), 958-64.

[35] Photocoagulation for diabetic macular edema Early Treatment Diabetic Retinopathy Study report number 1. Early Treatment Diabetic Retinopathy Study research group. *Arch Ophthalmol*, 1985, 103(12), 1796-806.

[36] Mitchell, P; Bandello, F; Schmidt-erfurth, U; et al. The RESTORE study, ranibizumab monotherapy or combined with laser versus laser monotherapy for diabetic macular edema *Ophthalmology*, 2011, 118(4), 615-25.

[37] Christoforidis, JB; D'Amico, DJ. Surgical and other treatments of diabetic macular edema: an update. *Int Ophthalmol Clin*, 2004, 44(1), 139-60.

[38] Misra, A; Bachmann, MO; Greenwood, RH; et al. Trends in yield and effects of screening intervals during 17 years of a large UK community-based diabetic retinopathy screening programme. *Diabet Med*, 2009, 26(10), 1040-7.

[39] Young, T; Palta, M; Dempsey, J; Peppard, PE; Nieto, FJ; Hla, KM. Burden of sleep apnea: rationale; design; and major findings of the Wisconsin Sleep Cohort study. *WMJ*, 2009, 108(5), 246-9.

[40] West, SD; Nicoll, DJ; Stradling, JR. Prevalence of obstructive sleep apnoea in men with type 2 diabetes *Thorax*, 2006, 61(11), 945-50.

[41] Foster, GD; Sanders, MH; Millman, R; et al. Obstructive sleep apnea among obese patients with type 2 diabetes *Diabetes Care*, 2009, 32(6), 1017-9.

[42] Pepperell, JC; Ramdassingh-dow, S; Crosthwaite, N; et al. Ambulatory blood pressure after therapeutic and subtherapeutic nasal continuous positive airway pressure for obstructive sleep apnoea: a randomised parallel trial *Lancet*, 2002, 359(9302), 204-10.

[43] Punjabi, NM; Sorkin, JD; Katzel, LI; Goldberg, AP; Schwartz, AR; Smith, PL. Sleep-disordered breathing and insulin resistance in middle-aged and overweight men. *Am J Respir Crit Care Med*, 2002, 165(5), 677-82.

[44] Marin, JM; Carrizo, SJ; Vicente, E; Agusti, AG. Long-term cardiovascular outcomes in men with obstructive sleep apnoea-hypopnoea with or without treatment with continuous positive airway pressure: an observational study. *Lancet*, 2005, 365(9464), 1046-53.

[45] West, SD; Groves, DC; Lipinski, HJ; et al. The prevalence of retinopathy in men with Type 2 diabetes and obstructive sleep apnoea. *Diabet Med*, 2010, 27(4), 423-30.

[46] Kosseifi, S; Bailey, B; Price, R; Roy, TM; Byrd, RP; Peiris, AN. The association between obstructive sleep apnea syndrome and microvascular complications in well-controlled diabetic patients *Mil Med*, 2010, 175(11), 913-6.

[47] Mason, RH; West, SD; Kiire, CA; et al. High prevalence of sleep disordered breathing in patients with diabetic macular edema *Retina* (Philadelphia, Pa) 2012, 32(9), 1791-8.

[48] Shiba, T; Sato, Y; Takahashi, M. Relationship between diabetic retinopathy and sleep-disordered breathing *Am J Ophthalmol*, 2009, 147(6), 1017-21.

[49] Shiba, T; Maeno, T; Saishin, Y; Hori, Y; Takahashi, M. Nocturnal intermittent serious hypoxia and reoxygenation in proliferative diabetic retinopathy cases. *Am J Ophthalmol*, 2010, 149(6), 959-63.

[50] Rudrappa, S; Warren, G; Idris, I. Obstructive sleep apnoea is associated with the development and progression of diabetic retinopathy, independent of conventional risk factors and novel biomarkers for diabetic retinopathy *Br J Ophthalmol*, 2012, 96(12), 1535.

[51] Zhang, R; Guo, X; Guo, L; Lu, J; Zhou, X; Ji, L. Prevalence and associated factors of obstructive sleep apnea in hospitalized patients with type 2 diabetes in Beijing; China 2. *J Diabetes*, 2015, 7(1), 16-23.

[52] Mason, RH; West, SD; Kiire, CA; et al. High prevalence of sleep disordered breathing in patients with diabetic macular edema *Retina* (Philadelphia, Pa) 2012, 32(9), 1791-8.

[53] Schmidt, AM; Hori, O; Chen, JX; et al. Advanced glycation endproducts interacting with their endothelial receptor induce expression of vascular cell adhesion molecule -1 (VCAM -1) in cultured human endothelial cells and in mice A potential mechanism for the accelerated vasculopathy of diabetes *J Clin Invest*, 1995, 96(3), 1395-403.

[54] Koya, D; King, GL. Protein kinase C activation and the development of diabetic complications *Diabetes*, 1998, 47(6), 859-66.

[55] Du, XL; Edelstein, D; Rossetti, L; et al. Hyperglycemia-induced mitochondrial superoxide overproduction activates the hexosamine pathway and induces plasminogen activator inhibitor -1 expression by increasing Sp1 glycosylation *Proc Natl Acad Sci USA,* 2000, 97(22), 12222-6.

[56] Gabbay, KH; Merola, LO; Field, RA. Sorbitol pathway: presence in nerve and cord with substrate accumulation in diabetes *Science*, 1966, 151(3707), 209-10.

[57] Brownlee, M. The pathobiology of diabetic complications: a unifying mechanism. *Diabetes*, 2005, 54(6), 1615-25.

[58] Baynes, JW. Role of oxidative stress in development of complications in diabetes *Diabetes*, 1991, 40(4), 405-12.

[59] Arden, GB; Sivaprasad, S. The pathogenesis of early retinal changes of diabetic retinopathy *Doc Ophthalmol*, 2012, 124(1), 15-26.

[60] Schulz, R; Hummel, C; Heinemann, S; Seeger, W; Grimminger, F. Serum levels of vascular endothelial growth factor are elevated in patients with obstructive sleep apnea and severe nighttime hypoxia *Am J Respir Crit Care Med*, 2002, 165(1), 67-70.

[61] Ohga, E; Nagase, T; Tomita, T; et al. Increased levels of circulating ICAM -1, VCAM -1, and L-selectin in obstructive sleep apnea syndrome *J Appl Physiol*, 1999, 87(1), 10-4.

[62] Nesmith, BL; Ihnen, M; Schaal, S. Poor responders to bevacizumab pharmacotherapy in age-related macular degeneration and in diabetic macular edema demonstrate increased risk for obstructive sleep apnea *Retina* (Philadelphia, Pa) 2014, 34(12), 2423-30.

[63] Kowluru, RA; Chan, PS. Oxidative stress and diabetic retinopathy Exp *Diabetes Res.*, 2007, 2007, 43603.

[64] Braun, RD; Linsenmeier, RA; Goldstick, TK. Oxygen consumption in the inner and outer retina of the cat. *Invest Ophthalmol Vis Sci*, 1995, 36(3), 542-54.
[65] Cringle, S; Yu, DY; Alder, V; Su, EN. Oxygen tension and blood flow in the retina of normal and diabetic rats. *Adv Exp Med Biol*, 1992, 317, 787-91.
[66] Harris, A; Arend, O; Danis, RP; Evans, D; Wolf, S; Martin, BJ. Hyperoxia improves contrast sensitivity in early diabetic retinopathy *Br J Ophthalmol*, 1996, 80(3), 209-13.
[67] Juen, S; Kieselbach, GF. Electrophysiological changes in juvenile diabetics without retinopathy *Arch Ophthalmol*, 1990, 108(3), 372-5.
[68] Dean, FM; Arden, GB; Dornhorst, A. Partial reversal of protan and tritan colour defects with inhaled oxygen in insulin dependent diabetic subjects. *Br J Ophthalmol*, 1997, 81(1), 27-30.
[69] Arden, GB. The absence of diabetic retinopathy in patients with retinitis pigmentosa: implications for pathophysiology and possible treatment *Br J Ophthalmol*, 2001, 85(3), 366-70.
[70] Lahdenranta, J; Pasqualini, R; Schlingemann, RO; et al. An anti-angiogenic state in mice and humans with retinal photoreceptor cell degeneration. *Proc Natl Acad Sci USA,* 2001, 98(18), 10368-73.
[71] Nguyen, QD; Shah, SM; Van anden, E; Sung, JU; Vitale, S; Campochiaro, PA. Supplemental oxygen improves diabetic macular edema: a pilot study *Invest Ophthalmol Vis Sci*, 2004, 45(2), 617-24.
[72] Arden, GB; Gündüz, MK; Kurtenbach, A; et al. A preliminary trial to determine whether prevention of dark adaptation affects the course of early diabetic retinopathy *Eye* (Lond) 2010, 24(7), 1149-55.
[73] Arden, GB; Jyothi, S; Hogg, CH; Lee, YF; Sivaprasad, S. Regression of early diabetic macular oedema is associated with prevention of dark adaptation *Eye* (Lond) 2011, 25(12), 1546-54.
[74] Mason, RH; Kiire, CA; Groves, DC; et al. Visual improvement following continuous positive airway pressure therapy in diabetic subjects with clinically significant macular oedema and obstructive sleep apnoea: proof of principle study. *Respiration*, 2012, 84(4), 275-82.

In: Eye Diseases ...
Editor: Mingwu Wang

ISBN: 978-1-63482-894-9

Chapter 8

Glaucoma and Sleep Disorders

Clara M. Choo, MD and Patrick L. Tsai*, MD, MHA
Department of Ophthalmology and Vision Science,
University of Arizona College of Medicine, AZ, US

Case Presentation

A 54-year old obese Hispanic man presents to the clinic. The patient complains of occasional foreign body sensation and tearing, and has a brother who uses eye drops for glaucoma On exam, the upper eyelids are easily everted and the cornea has some punctate epithelial erosions. Intraocular pressures are slightly above normal at 24 mm Hg in each eye and the optic nerve cup to disc ratio is 0.7. A glaucoma work-up is ordered, including visual fields and optic nerve photos, and the patient is told to return to clinic in 1 month for an intraocular pressure check, optical coherence tomography, and a second baseline visual field. In the meantime, the patient is started on ocular lubrication for his floppy eyelid syndrome and referred to primary care for a sleep study and sleep apnea evaluation.

* E-mail: ptsai@eyes.arizona.edu.

Glaucoma: An Overview

Glaucoma is a class of diseases marked by a progressive optic neuropathy with a typical excavation pattern that leads to visual field loss. It is a multifactorial disease that can be characterized into 1) open versus closed angle, referring to the nature of the aqueous outflow path, and 2) primary and secondary causes, where there are identifiable anatomical anomalies creating an outflow obstruction.

The aqueous outflow pathway begins at the ciliary body, the site of aqueous humor production. The fluid then moves through the posterior chamber between the lens and the iris forward into the anterior chamber. The aqueous is drained by the trabecular meshwork into Schlemm's canal-episcleral venous system and the alternate uveoscleral outflow pathway. [1] Conventional outflow through the trabecular meshwork is a function of both the contractile properties of the meshwork in addition to the osmolarity of the aqueous. A hypoosmolar aqueous has been correlated to swelling in meshwork cell volume, decreasing outflow facility. The nonconventional uveoscleral pathway is dependent on the contractile properties of the ciliary body muscle; the more relaxed the muscle, the greater aqueous flow through the ciliary muscle (Figure 1). [1]

In the open angle glaucoma class, which includes primary open angle glaucoma, normal tension glaucoma and ocular hypertension among other diagnoses, there is no known physical blockage of the aqueous outflow system. The obstruction is thought to be secondary to an increased resistance of the trabecular meshwork's extracellular matrix and trabecular cells. Normal tension glaucoma is a type of open angle glaucoma where glaucomatous damage occurs in the setting of physiologic pressures. Ocular hypertension, on the other hand, is persistently elevated intraocular pressure (IOP), in the absence of any documented nerve damage.

In angle closure glaucoma, the aqueous outflow path may be obstructed among several different points along the normal pathway. For instance, in primary angle closure glaucoma with pupillary block, iris-lens contact restricts aqueous movement from the posterior to anterior chamber leading to forward iris bowing and narrowing of the iridocorneal angle (Figure 2). Plateau iris configuration can also lead to angle closure. Moreover, angle closure can occur due to the angle being closed by peripheral anterior synechiae, scar-like tissue spanning across the iridocorneal angle, or a posterior pushing mechanism, like a posterior segment tumor moving the lens-iris complex anteriorly.

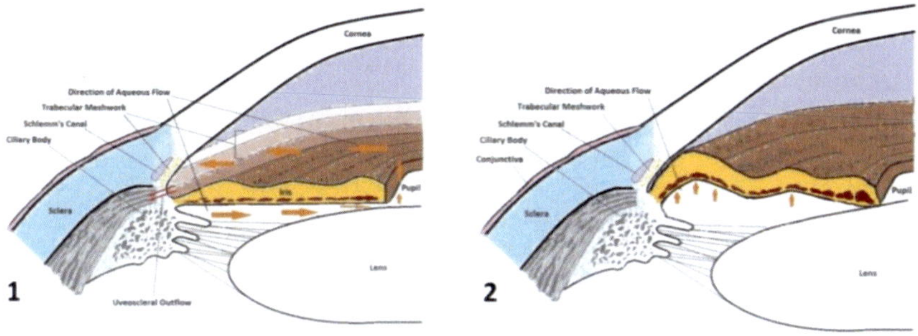

Figure 1. Normal and open angle configuration Aqueous humor is produced at the ciliary body. Conventional flow (trabecular meshwork-Schlemm's canal-episcleral venous system) is demonstrated with orange arrows, with the nonconventional uveoscleral pathway noted with red arrows. In open angle glaucoma, although there are no major angle changes, there is increased resistance to flow at the trabecular meshwork. Figure 2. Closed angle configuration with pupillary block. Aqueous humor is produced at the ciliary body. Due to pupillary block, the aqueous cannot travel from the posterior to anterior chamber. Posterior chamber pressure pushes the peripheral iris forward to crowd the iridocorneal angle. (Illustration by Mingwu Wang, MD, PhD)

Primary glaucomas are not associated with any known eye or other systemic diseases, whereas secondary glaucomas are linked with an underlying disorder. For instance, secondary open angle glaucomas include diseases where there is increased resistance at the trabecular meshwork from a deposition of material, such as pigments in pigment dispersion syndrome. In secondary angle closure glaucomas, angle closure may occur due to an anterior pulling or posterior pushing mechanism, like chronic inflammation causing scar tissue formation along the iridocorneal angle or neovascularization covering the angle.

Primary open angle glaucoma is found in approximately 2 percent of the US adults above the age of 40, a total of 2.2 million people affected. Worldwide, incidence is estimated at about 2.4 million persons per year, with about 4 million people with bilateral blindness. [2] It is the second most common cause of blindness after cataracts. In the early stage of the disease, it is often asymptomatic. As retinal ganglion cell loss progresses, peripheral visual field loss may advance to central vision decline.

High IOP is a major risk factor for the disease, but it is neither necessary nor sufficient in the diagnosis of the disease. Currently, topical medical therapies are aimed at lowering intraocular pressure Other commonly recognized risk factors for glaucoma include advanced age, family history, race (of African and Hispanic descent), and low central corneal thickness.

In cases where IOP is within the normal range (generally 10-22 mm Hg), but there is documented nerve loss, it is believed that patients' threshold for nerve damage is lower than typical glaucoma cases. This is known as normal tension glaucoma, and generally is managed and treated similarly to open angle glaucoma The IOP that these eyes tolerate without sustaining damage is on the lower end of normal.

Primary angle closure glaucoma has a prevalence of about 0.1 percent among the Caucasian American population, but it is thought to be as high as 2-4 percent in Inuit and Asians. Other risk factors for narrow angle glaucoma include female gender, age, hyperopic eyes and family history, all of which are linked to more shallow anterior chamber depth Symptoms can vary according to the time frame of onset. Acute angle closure attacks where there is a large change in IOP over a matter of hours can cause red eye, eye pain, halos, nausea and vomiting In contrast, chronic angle closure over weeks to months may cause a slow, asymptomatic elevation in the pressure.

The genetic and environmental contribution to the development of glaucoma is still being defined. Most of the genes that have been identified are transmitted in an autosomal dominant pattern with incomplete penetrance GLC1A, a trabecular meshwork glucocorticoid gene, is found in 3 percent of the POAG population. [3] Other loci of the GL1 gene have been implicated to a lesser degree. A positive sibling history can confer risk for glaucoma (10 percent prevalence). However, twin studies have shown that monozygotic pairs have only a slightly higher concordance for POAG (10.3 percent) than dizygotic pairs (1.3 percent), suggesting the importance of environmental influences. [4]

In the clinical setting, glaucoma is diagnosed and managed by taking into account several factors. During the first evaluation, a pertinent history may include general medical history and systemic medication use (beta agonists, beta blocker s, steroids, anti-seizure medications), family history of glaucoma or systemic disorders associated with secondary forms of glaucoma, and history of trauma A full eye exam will include best-corrected visual acuity with refraction, pupil examination, confrontational fields, gonioscopy, tonometry, pachymetry, anterior segment and dilated posterior segment evaluation. Gonioscopy is the examination of the iridocorneal angle, where the primary aqueous outflow pathway lies. The angle is graded on the angle width (0 to 45 degrees), the apparent insertion of the iris to the iridocorneal angle structures and the iris' spatial position. Tonometry is the measurement of IOP, whereas pachymetry is the measurement of the central corneal thickness, which can help extrapolate risk of primary open angle glaucoma.

The posterior segment exam is crucial to the assessment of the optic nerve under an optimal stereoscopic view. The optic nerve is evaluated on the cup to disc ratio, both in the horizontal and vertical meridians. Color and contour of the nerve is also documented, with close attention to areas of pallor and neural rim thinning or sloping. The orientation of blood vessels emanating from the optic nerve also provides clues to the configuration of the optic nerve (Figure 3). If areas of thinning or sloping are noted that correlate with other signs of damage found on the visual fields or optical coherence tomography (OCT), this increases suspicion that the damage is non-physiologic and real. Flame-shaped disc hemorrhages perpendicular to the disc margin, also known as Drance hemorrhages, can signal progression of glaucoma tous disease. The exact mechanism of their formation, while still uncertain, may be the result of shearing of blood vessels caused by altered blood flow at the lamina cribrosa secondary to neurodegeneration Others have postulated that a primary vascular etiology may be to blame. [2]

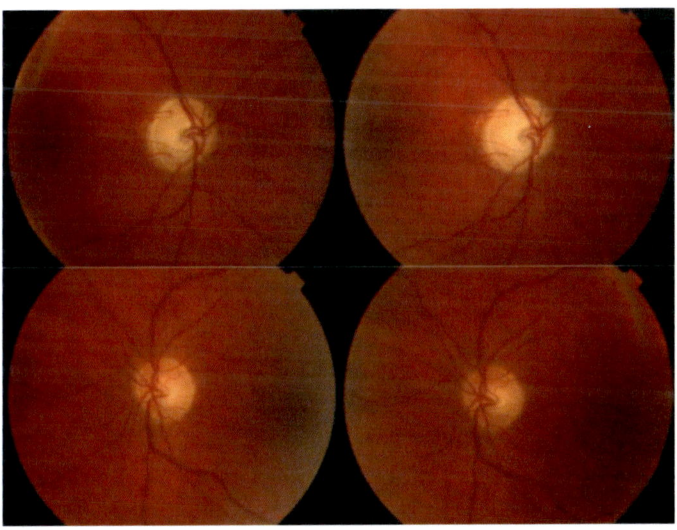

Figure 3. Stereoscopic disc photos. Right eye (above) shows a cup to disc ratio of 0.7 with inferior thinning (note the sloping of vessels). Left eye (below) demonstrates a cup to disc ratio of 0.5 with an even rim of nerve fiber layer tissue.

Ancillary testing is critical to the diagnosis and long-term management of glaucoma. Visual field testing (VFT) can quantify the quality of peripheral vision in comparison to age-matched normals. This can be followed over time to see if there are characteristic signs of glaucomatous damage, which can include a nasal step, a superior (Figure 4) or inferior arcuate pattern (which follows the retinal ganglion cell radiations), or a paracentral scotoma. If there is a cluster of three or more damaged points that persists on repeated testing, this can be especially telling of glaucoma damage.

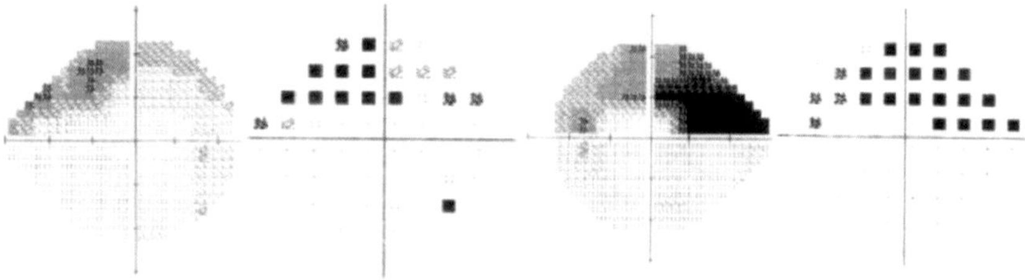

Figure 4. Humphrey visual fields with grayscale and total deviation diagrams of the right and left eye. Both eyes demonstrate a superior arcuate defect, which is denser in the left eye. The total deviation plots show the tested points on the field that stray from normal age-matched controls.

Equally important in glaucoma assessment is the thickness of nerve fiber layer (NFL) provided by OCT. This is a non-invasive technique that uses low coherence interferometry to calculate delay in echo time and the amount of light reflected off a target object. This is like an ultrasound, but using light waves instead of sound waves. As with visual field testing, a single patient's nerve fiber layer is compared with an age-matched database and rated on its thickness. Areas of glaucoma damage typically start in the superior or inferior portions of the nerve (Figure 5). Often times the thinning of the optic NFL detected by OCT will herald visual field changes.

Current medical management of glaucoma is primarily directed at lowering intraocular pressure, either by decreasing production of aqueous humor at the ciliary body or by increasing drainage through the trabecular meshwork or through uveoscleral outflow. Topical alpha agonists both decrease production and increases trabecular outflow. Topical beta blockers and carbonic anhydrase inhibitors decrease aqueous production. Systemic forms of beta blockers and carbonic anhydrase inhibitors have been found to lower intraocular pressure, but are typically not prescribed for a primary glaucoma condition. Prostaglandin analogs increase outflow through the uveoscleral pathway. Topical cholinergic eye drops are infrequently used mainly to manage closed-angle glaucoma to cause pupillary constriction and increase trabecular outflow. If medical management is insufficient, laser and incisional surgeries may be necessary.

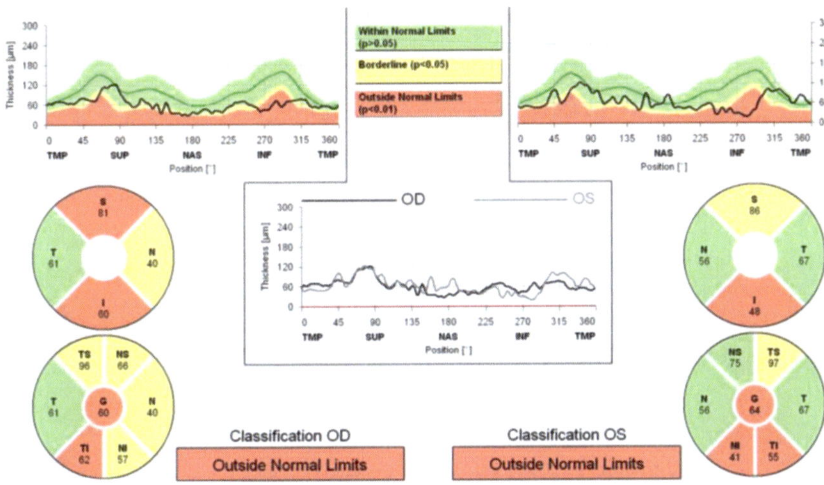

Figure 5. Optical coherence tomography demonstrating inferior and superior nerve fiber layer thinning with borderline nasal thinning of the right eye, and inferior thinning with superior borderline thinning of the left eye.

Laser trabeculoplasty is the application of laser energy to the trabecular meshwork. It may cause local shrinkage leading to areas of stretched trabecular meshwork. However, the leading theory for selective laser trabeculoplasty is that interleukin-1B and tumor necrosis factor-alpha are released to stimulate matrix metalloproteinases which increase outflow facility. Intraocular pressure lowering by laser trabeculoplasty is modest, around 20-25 percent. This effect can last 6-12 months in 80 percent of patients, 3-5 years in 50 percent of patients, and 10 years in 30 percent of patients. [5]

The two main surgical interventions for open angle glaucomas are trabeculectomy and glaucoma drainage device implantation. In a trabeculectomy, a partial thickness scleral window is made adjacent to the corneoscleral junction to increase outflow facility into a filtering bleb. When glaucoma drainage devices are implanted into the eye, a tube is placed directly into the iridocorneal angle to allow aqueous to drain directly from the anterior chamber into a subconjunctival space. Success rates and complications can be variable depending on technique, thus surgical intervention is typically recommended after maximal medical therapy and laser treatments have been tried first.

In angle closure glaucoma s, an alternate aqueous flow pathway can be achieved with laser iridotomy or surgical peripheral iridectomy. In both procedures, peripheral iris tissue is removed to allow aqueous to travel from the posterior to anterior chamber without passing through the iris lens diaphragm.

The progressive loss of retinal ganglion cells in open or closed angle glaucomas is still being studied. As IOP reduction is the major modifiable risk factor, direct compression of the nerve and its effects on the hemodynamic supply is implicated. One theory is that the compression of the nerve at the lamina cribrosa causes a disruption of axoplasmic flow. [6] It may also alter the nerve's ability to autoregulate blood supply to itself, leading to optic nerve damage. Other proposed mechanisms include oxidative injury and glutamate toxicity seen in diseases like Parkinson's and Alzheimer's diseases. [7]

Normal Physiologic Changes of IOP in Sleep and the Circadian Rhythm of the Eye

In normal subjects, blood pressure typically dips about 10-20 percent from daytime values. Subjects that have higher or lower than normal nocturnal blood pressure dips have an increased association with ischemic phenomena, including myocardial infection, stroke, and other thrombotic and hemorrhagic events. The ocular perfusion pressure is calculated by subtracting the intraocular pressure from the mean arterial pressure (OPP= MAP-IOP). In glaucoma, both the MAP and the IOP are theorized to be affected. A greater nocturnal blood pressure dip and higher nocturnal intraocular pressures lead to higher fluctuations of ocular perfusion pressure, which have been associated with glaucomatous field changes. [8] However, there are conflicting studies whether ocular perfusion pressure is increased or decreased during sleep and further investigation is needed.

IOP measurements during a 24-hour period reveal a diurnal variation, up to 2-6 mm Hg in normal subjects and up to 10 mm Hg in subjects with glaucoma. [2, 9] Under sleep laboratory conditions, the highest IOP recordings occur at nighttime and are likely not captured during routine eye examinations

The definitive relationship between IOP fluctuation and optic nerve damage is yet unknown.

Aqueous humor secretion also fluctuates during a 24-hour cycle. Aqueous humor secretion rates are higher during the daytime and lower at nighttime, about half the daytime rate. In sleep deprivation lab conditions, the secretion rate is elevated above normal nighttime rates but still below typical daytime secretion. [2] The hormones responsible for the circadian rhythm of aqueous production include epinephrine and cortisol, with melatonin and serotonin also possibly playing a role. The adrenal gland secretes epinephrine and cortisol, both of which have a nocturnal dip. [10]

Melatonin is a crucial sleep hormone, and is produced in the retina and ciliary body in addition to the pineal gland. [11] Upstream to the production of melatonin are the intrinsically photosensitive retinal ganglion cells (ipRGCs, a subset of RGCs), which releases melanopsin. Melanopsin sends feedback to the suprachiasmatic nucleus, located in the hypothalamus above the optic chiasm to regulate the light-dark cycle, the pupillary light reflex and melatonin secretion Melatonin interacts with G-protein coupled receptors that downregulate adenylatecyclase. There are two receptor subtypes, MT1 and MT2, found in the uvea and the retina. [12]

In further support of the importance of melatonin, animal models of glaucoma have demonstrated degeneration of ipRGC and a decrease in melanopsin pigment. When melatonin was injected in wild type mice, IOP decreased significantly. However, in knockout mice lacking the melatonin receptor type 1 and type 2, there was no change in IOP. [13] In knockout mice lacking the melatonin receptor type 1, higher nocturnal IOPs were noted and numbers of retinal ganglion cells reduced by up to 25-30 percent. In contrast, melatonin receptor type 2 knockouts did not show any differences in IOP or RGCs. [12] It was hypothesized that melatonin acts on G-protein coupled receptors to down regulate adenylatecyclase, thereby decreasing aqueous humor production at the ciliary body and reducing oxidative stress experienced by RGCs. Furthermore, another knockout mice study demonstrated fewer retinal ganglion cells at 18 months. [14] The role of melatonin as a neuroprotector is still being investigated, but in human studies topical melatonin has been shown to decrease IOP. [15]

Serotonin is another important neuroregulator that can modulate sleep, mood, hunger and pain. [16] Within the eye, a diverse subset of receptors is found in the cornea, sclera, iris, ciliary body and retina Topical serotonin in rabbit models has been found to increase IOP, [17] possibly by increasing the ciliary body blood flow and thus increasing aqueous production. [16, 18]

Systemic and topical application of serotonin type-2 receptor antagonist ketanserin has lowered IOP in controls and glaucoma patients. [19] With the use of selective serotonin receptor inhibitors to treat depression and other psychiatric disorders, there have been several case studies of patients with IOP elevations manifesting as acute angle closure glaucoma attacks. [20-25] In addition to the above mechanisms, serotonin type 5 receptor may induce smooth muscle relaxation at the iris sphincter, leading to mydriasis [23-25] as well as cAMP elevation leading to increased aqueous humor production.

Glaucoma and Obstructive Sleep Apnea

Some authors have suggested the monitoring of IOP on a 24-hour basis if the therapeutic IOP goal has not been met. However, it should be noted that measurement of IOP in the upright position in office may not accurately reflect IOP experienced during sleep There have been many studies pointing to the correlation of glaucoma tous damage with obstructive sleep apnea (OSA) Although several theoretical mechanisms have been suggested in the literature, none have been definitively elucidated. Glaucoma and OSA share common risk factors such as advanced age and an association with cardiovascular disease One study found that there was a 7.2 percent prevalence of glaucoma in the OSA population, compared with 2 percent in the general population. [26] Furthermore, the authors concluded that the amount of glaucoma damage (optic nerve changes and visual field losses) positively correlated with the respiratory disturbance index (RDI = apnea s/hour). This has been supported by other studies, [27-29] although there are contrary reports suggesting there is no correlation between RDI and IOP/glaucoma damage. [30-32]

In a prospective cohort study, [33] 1012 patients with an OSA diagnosis were followed for the development of open angle glaucoma over a 5-year period. They found that the risk ratio was 1.67, or about a 5.6 percent development rate, in comparison to the controls without OSA with a 3.4 percent rate over the same period. Hypertension, diabetes, chronic kidney disease, obesity and hyperlipidemia, and socioeconomic status were accounted for; OSA was found to be an independent risk factor in the development of glaucoma.

The exact mechanism of how OSA affects glaucoma is not known, but it likely has to do with the changing hemodynamics within the body that results in altered blood flow to the eye. The hypoxia, hypercapnia and inspiratory effort cause fluctuations in oxygen and carbon dioxide levels beyond the optic nerve head's ability to autoregulate flow. As mentioned previously, glaucoma patients have been found to have lower nocturnal systemic blood pressures and higher IOPs, leading to lower ocular perfusion pressure s. Positioning during sleep can significantly increase the IOPs on the dependent eye. The IOPs recorded in the neck flexion/extension, supine and lateral decubitus positions are higher than the sitting position. Moreover, elevating the head of the bed by 30 degrees will lower IOP by up to 20 percent in comparison to the supine position. [34] Another study found that recorded supine IOPs and the IOP from a change in posture did negatively correlate to the change in mean deviation of visual fields when followed for at least 2 years. [9]

Furthermore, the hypoxemia, hypercapnia and increased inspiratory effort in OSA can lead to a decrease in ocular perfusion pressure Obstruction from the loss of normal upper airway tone or narrowing of the soft palate is associated with at least a 30 percent airflow reduction and at least 4 percent oxygen desaturation. [35] This disrupts the ability for the optic nerve to autoregulate blood flow during prolonged periods of apnea s. Arteriosclerosis and an imbalance between vasodilator nitric oxide and vasoconstrictor endothelin can also contribute to the dysregulation. [33] Interestingly, in the management of glaucoma, calcium channel blocks act as a vasodilator to improve vascular supply to the optic disc and this particular form of systemic hypertensive treatment has been suggested. [36, 37]

Additionally, the disruption of normal sleep patterns in OSA has been shown to have a detrimental effect on melatonin levels. Elevated nocturnal norepinephrine levels in OSA patients have been correlated with melatonin release. [38, 39] The diminished nocturnal melatonin levels could result in higher IOPs. This would subsequently lower ocular perfusion pressures and result in greater glaucoma tous damage and progression. One study found that the normal nocturnal peak of melatonin was diminished in these patients. Adding continuous positive airway pressure (CPAP) treatment actually decreased the amount of melatonin in circulation on first treatment day, presumably by decreasing the sympathetic stimulus. [40] Further studies would be needed to track long-term effects of CPAP use on melatonin levels. The long-term effects of CPAP on the eye have yet to be studied. One study citing worsened NFL damage with more severe OSA cases suggests that CPAP treatment may prevent visual field damage. [41] However, a different prospective study demonstrated an increase in intraocular pressure in sleep apnea patients after they had initiated CPAP treatment. [42] Some other CPAP related complications to the eye include dry eye syndrome, bacterial conjunctivitis and limbal keratitis. [35] Finally, the effect of surgical and combined CPAP/surgical interventions has been shown to slightly decrease the hazard ratio in the development of glaucoma. [43]

At the very least, the presence of a glaucoma diagnosis and sleep symptoms consistent with OSA should prompt the eyecare providers to suggest further investigation such as a sleep study. Primary care providers should also consider sending their patients with sleep disorders for eye screening exams, as oftentimes glaucoma is an insidious disease that can be asymptomatic at onset and requires careful monitoring.

Glaucoma and Other Sleep Disorders

There is less evidence for a relationship between other sleep disorders (besides OSA) and glaucoma (besides open angle glaucoma), but there are published subjective studies among patients with glaucoma. When surveyed, patients with moderate to high visual field defects due to open angle glaucoma tended to report a higher sleep disturbance pattern (for instance, a longer time to fall asleep) than those with none to minimal visual field defects. [44] The authors postulate that the impaired rise in melatonin in the setting of glaucoma could lead to an altered circadian rhythm. [45] It is also possible that an impairment in melatonin release as part of an impaired circadian rhythm leads to the increased glaucoma damage.

Furthermore, in a survey of patients with open and closed angle glaucoma, the prevalence of sleep disturbance was as high as 81 percent in angle closure patients, compared to 47 percent of open angle patients and 23 percent of control patients. [11] Interestingly, no correlation was found between the highest recorded IOP, day or night, and the amount of sleep disturbance reported. Why would there be a difference in the severity of sleep disturbance between open and closed angle glaucoma? One hypothesis is that over time, an eye with chronically closed angle will experience higher average IOPs than one with chronically open angle. As a result, instead of the intrinsically photosensitive retinal ganglion cells being selectively damaged, both ipRGCs and upstream photoreceptors sustain damage. With less input from photoreceptors, the limited numbers of ipRGCs have less stimuli to secrete melanopsin. Alternatively, there may be receptors within the trabecular meshwork that are inhibited by the lack of aqueous flow in closed angle glaucoma. This inhibition may prevent the release of neurotransmitters or neuropeptides that may feedback to control IOP regulation and circadian rhythms.

References

[1] Llobet, A; Gasull, X; Gual, A. Understanding trabecular meshwork physiology: a key to the control of intraocular pressure? *News Physiol Sci*, 2003, 18, 205-9.

[2] American Academy of Ophthalmology. Basic and Clinical Science Course, Glaucoma, Section 10, 2013-2014. San Francisco, 2013.

[3] Stone, EM; Fingert, JH; Alward, WL; Nguyen, TD; Polansky, JR; Sunden, SL; et al. Identification of a gene that causes primary open angle glaucoma. *Science*, 1997, 275(5300), 668-70.

[4] Teikari, JM; Kaprio, J; Koskenvuo, M; Vannas, A. Ophthalmic disease in twins: a nationwide record linkage study of hospital discharges and free medications for 16,067 twin pairs. *Acta Genet Med Gemellol (Roma)*, 1987, 36(4), 523-34.

[5] Mitrev, P; Schuman, J. Lasers in glaucoma management Focal Points: Clinical Modules for Ophthalmologists. San Francisco: American Academy of Ophthalmology, 2001.

[6] Mackenzie, PJ; Cioffi, GA. Vascular anatomy of the optic nerve head. *Can J Ophthalmol*, 2008, 43(3), 308-12.

[7] Gupta, N; Yucel, YH. Glaucoma as a neurodegenerative disease. *Curr Opin Ophthalmol*, 2007, 18(2), 110-4.

[8] Aref, AA. What happens to glaucoma patients during sleep? *Curr Opin Ophthalmol*, 2013, 24(2), 162-6.

[9] Kiuchi, T; Motoyama, Y; Oshika, T. Relationship of progression of visual field damage to postural changes in intraocular pressure in patients with normal-tension glaucoma *Ophthalmology*, 2006, 113(12), 2150-5.

[10] Gherghel, D; Hosking, SL; Orgul, S. Autonomic nervous system, circadian rhythm s, and primary open-angle glaucoma *Surv Ophthalmol*, 2004, 49(5), 491-508.

[11] Wang, H; Zhang, Y; Ding, J; Wang, N. Changes in the circadian rhythm in patients with primary glaucoma *PLoS One*, 2013, 8(4), e62841.

[12] Tosini, G; Iuvone, M; Boatright, JH. Is the melatonin receptor type 1 involved in the pathogenesis of glaucoma? *J Glaucoma*, 2013, 22 Suppl 5, S49-50.

[13] Alcantara-Contreras, S; Baba, K; Tosini, G. Removal of melatonin receptor type 1 increases intraocular pressure and retinal ganglion cells death in the mouse. *Neurosci Lett*, 2011, 494(1), 61-4.

[14] Baba, K; Pozdeyev, N; Mazzoni, F; Contreras-Alcantara, S; Liu, C; Kasamatsu, M; et al. Melatonin modulates visual function and cell viability in the mouse retina via the MT1 melatonin receptor. *Proc Natl Acad Sci U S A*, 2009, 106(35), 15043-8.

[15] Samples, JR; Krause, G; Lewy, AJ. Effect of melatonin on intraocular pressure *Curr Eye Res*, 1988, 7(7), 649-53.

[16] Costagliola, C; Parmeggiani, F; Semeraro, F; Sebastiani, A. Selective serotonin reuptake inhibitors: a review of its effects on intraocular pressure *Curr Neuropharmacol*, 2008, 6(4), 293-310.

[17] Mallorga, P; Sugrue, MF. Characterization of serotonin receptors in the iris + ciliary body of the albino rabbit. *Curr Eye Res*, 1987, 6(3), 527-32.

[18] Costagliola, C; Mastropasqua, L; Capone, D; Verolino, M; Ciancaglini, M; Pisanti, N. Effect of fluoxetine on intraocular pressure in the rabbit. *Exp Eye Res*, 2000, 70(5), 551-5.

[19] Mastropasqua, L; Ciancaglini, M; Carpineto, P; Costagliola, C. Ocular hypotensive effect of topical ketanserin in timolol users. *Graefes Arch Clin Exp Ophthalmol*, 1997, 235(3), 130-5.

[20] Ahmad, S. Fluoxetine and glaucoma *DICP*, 1991, 25(4), 436.

[21] Browning, AC; Reck, AC; Chisholm, IH; Nischal, KK. Acute angle closure glaucoma presenting in a young patient after administration of paroxetine *Eye* (*Lond*), 2000, 14(Pt 3A), 406-8.

[22] Levy, J; Tessler, Z; Klemperer, I; Shneck, M; Lifshitz, T. Late bilateral acute angle-closure glaucoma after administration of paroxetine in a patient with plateau iris configuration *Can J Ophthalmol*, 2004, 39(7), 780-1.

[23] Eke, T; Bates, AK. Acute angle closure glaucoma associated with paroxetine *BMJ* 1997, 314(7091), 1387.

[24] Kirwan, JF; Subak-Sharpe, I; Teimory, M. Bilateral acute angle closure glaucoma after administration of paroxetine *Br J Ophthalmol*, 1997, 81(3), 252.

[25] Lewis, CF; DeQuardo, JR; DuBose, C; Tandon, R. Acute angle-closure glaucoma and paroxetine *J Clin Psychiatry*, 1997, 58(3), 123-4.

[26] Mojon, DS; Hess, CW; Goldblum, D; Fleischhauer, J; Koerner, F; Bassetti, C; et al. High prevalence of glaucoma in patients with sleep apnea syndrome *Ophthalmology*, 1999, 106(5), 1009-12.

[27] Tsang, CS; Chong, SL; Ho, CK; Li, MF. Moderate to severe obstructive sleep apnoea patients is associated with a higher incidence of visual field defect. *Eye* (*Lond*), 2006, 20(1), 38-42.

[28] Mojon, DS; Mathis, J; Zulauf, M; Koerner, F; Hess, CW. Optic neuropathy associated with sleep apnea syndrome *Ophthalmology*, 1998, 105(5), 874-7.

[29] Zengin, MO; Tuncer, I; Karahan, E. Retinal nerve fiber layer thickness changes in obstructive sleep apnea syndrome: one year follow-up results. *Int J Ophthalmol*, 7(4), 704-8.

[30] Geyer, O; Cohen, N; Segev, E; Rath, EZ; Melamud, L; Peled, R; et al. The prevalence of glaucoma in patients with sleep apnea syndrome: same as in the general population *Am J Ophthalmol*, 2003, 136(6), 1093-6.

[31] Aptel, F; Chiquet, C; Tamisier, R; Sapene, M; Martin, F; Stach, B; et al. Association between glaucoma and sleep apnea in a large French multicenter prospective cohort. *Sleep Med*, 15(5), 576-81.

[32] Khandgave, TP; Puthran, N; Ingole, AB; Nicholson, AD The assessment of sleep apnoea as a risk factor in glaucoma *J Clin DiagnRes*, 7(7), 1391-3.

[33] Lin, CC; Hu, CC; Ho, JD; Chiu, HW; Lin, HC. Obstructive sleep apnea and increased risk of glaucoma: a population-based matched-cohort study. *Ophthalmology*, 2013, 120(8), 1559-64.

[34] Malihi, M; Sit, AJ. Effect of head and body position on intraocular pressure *Ophthalmology*, 2012, 119(5), 987-91.

[35] Waller, EA; Bendel, RE; Kaplan, J. Sleep disorders and the eye. *Mayo Clin Proc*, 2008, 83(11), 1251-61.

[36] Kitazawa, Y; Shirai, H; Go, FJ. The effect of Ca2(+) -antagonist on visual field in low-tension glaucoma *Graefes Arch Clin Exp Ophthalmol*, 1989, 227(5), 408-12.

[37] Netland, PA; Chaturvedi, N; Dreyer, EB. Calcium channel blockers in the management of low-tension and open-angle glaucoma *Am J Ophthalmol*, 1993, 115(5), 608-13.

[38] Elmasry, A; Lindberg, E; Hedner, J; Janson, C; Boman, G. Obstructive sleep apnoca and urine catecholamines in hypertensive males: a population-based study. *Eur Respir J*, 2002, 19(3), 511-7.

[39] Heitmann, J; Ehlenz, K; Penzel, T; Becker, HF; Grote, L; Voigt, KH; et al. Sympathetic activity is reduced by nCPAP in hypertensive obstructive sleep apnoea patients. *Eur Respir J*, 2004, 23(2), 255-62.

[40] Hernandez, C; Abreu, J; Abreu, P; Castro, A; Jimenez, A. Nocturnal melatonin plasma levels in patients with OSAS:the effect of CPAP. *Eur Respir J*, 2007, 30(3), 496-500.

[41] Lin, PW; Friedman, M; Lin, HC; Chang, HW; Wilson, M; Lin, MC. Normal tension glaucoma in patients with obstructive sleep apnea /hypopnea syndrome *J Glaucoma*, 2011, 20(9), 553-8.

[42] Kiekens, S; VevaDe, G; Coeckelbergh, T; Tassignon, MJ; vande, Heyning, P; Wilfried, De, B; et al. Continuous positive airway pressure therapy is associated with an increase in intraocular pressure in obstructive sleep apnea *Invest Ophthalmol Vis Sci*, 2008, 49(3), 934-40.

[43] Chen, HY; Chang, YC; Lin, CC; Sung, FC; Chen, WC. Obstructive sleep apnea patients having surgery are less associated with glaucoma *J Ophthalmol*, 2014, 838912.

[44] Agorastos, A; Skevas, C; Matthaei, M; Otte, C; Klemm, M; Richard, G; et al. Depression, anxiety, and disturbed sleep in glaucoma *J Neuropsychiatry Clin Neurosci*, 2013, 25(3), 205-13.

[45] Srinivasan, V; Pandi-Perumal, SR; Trahkt, I; Spence, DW; Poeggeler, B; Hardeland, R; et al. Melatonin and melatonergic drugs on sleep, possible mechanisms of action. *Int J Neurosci*, 2009, 119(6), 821-46.

In: Eye Diseases …
Editor: Mingwu Wang

ISBN: 978-1-63482-894-9

Chapter 9

Papilledema and Sleep Disorders

Jane Cho, MD, and Le Yu**, *MD
Department of Ophthalmology and Vision Science,
University of Arizona College of Medicine, AZ, US

Case Presentation

A 35 years old obese female presents to clinic with a chief complaint of intermittent blurry vision in both eyes. A recent refraction improved her vision to 20/30 in each eye. Overall her past medical history is relatively benign except for chronic daily headaches of several years without recent change. Her husband relays his concern for her daytime excessive sleepiness, which has worsened during the past year. He cannot comment specifically on her sleep pattern at night because they reside in separate bedrooms due to her loud snoring. Pupillary exam shows mildly sluggish reaction to light in both eyes without the appearance of an afferent pupillary defect. A dilated fundus exam reveals bilateral disc edema with peripapillary hemorrhages (Figure 1). To work up the etiology of papilledema, a brain MRI /MRV is ordered, which is unremarkable. A subsequent lumbar puncture reveals an opening pressure of 340 mm H_2O and normal cerebral spinal fluid, confirming a diagnosis of papilledema due to elevated intracranial pressure.

* Email: lyu@eyes.arizona.edu.

Papilledema: An Overview

Papilledema is a term to describe optic disc swelling in the setting of increased intracranial pressure (ICP), which may be associated with a variety of conditions (e.g., intracranial lesions, masses, obstructive hydrocephalus, cerebral venous sinus thrombosis). When a cause for increased ICP cannot be found, it is referred to as idiopathic intracranial hypertension (IIH). It is a diagnosis of exclusion that meets the modified Dandy criteria, which includes an alert and awake patient with symptoms of increased ICP without localizing neurological signs, normal brain imaging results, ICP of more than 250 mm H_2O with normal cerebral spinal fluid (CSF) findings, and no identifiable cause of increased ICP. [1]

Regardless of the cause of papilledema, elevated ICP is believed to be transmitted to the eye through the optic nerve sheath resulting in subsequent mechanical disruption of axoplasmic flow within the optic nerve and swelling of the optic axons. This leads to a leakage of water, protein, and other cellular contents into the extracellular space within the optic nerve. [2] In the acute setting, the optic nerve appears hyperemic due to congestion of its microvascular flow with dilation and telangiectasia of the surface disc capillaries. Flame hemorrhages are frequently observed adjacent to the optic disc, and its margins and vessels are obscured due to edema of the peripapillary nerve fiber layer (Figure 1).

The absence of spontaneous venous pulsations is noted on clinical exam of all patients with acute papilledema as well as 20 percent of the normal population. [3] Grading the severity of papilledema is based on visual features of the optic disc and peripapillary retina. In addition, many ophthalmologists are now utilizing imaging modalities such as optic coherence tomography (OCT), a cross-sectional imaging technique that quantitatively assesses multiple layers of the retina using near-infrared light. Both OCT retinal nerve fiber layer (RNLF) thickness and total retinal thickness are found to be increased in patients with papilledema and generally these findings can be correlated with the clinical appearance of the nerve. [4]

In cases of chronic papilledema, the disc loses its hyperemic color and takes on a pale appearance from long-term axonal loss. Gliosis of the peripapillary nerve fiber layer occurs as the tissue appears less fluffy or edematous and more membranous (Figure 2).

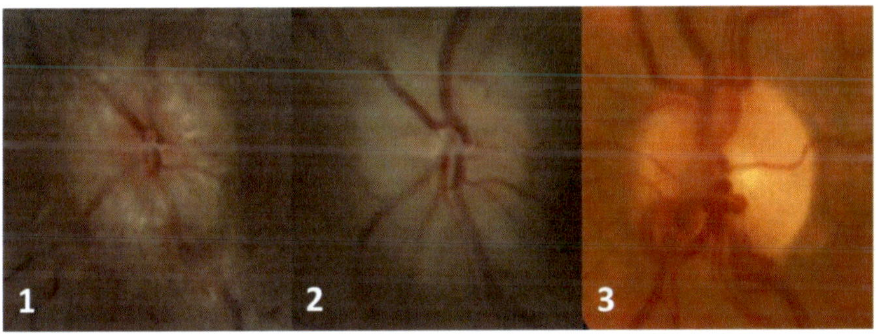

Figure 1. Acute papilledema with peripapillary flame hemorrhages and obscured optic disc margins and vessels. Figure 2. Chronic papilledema with optic disc pallor and gliosis of the peripapillary nerve fiber layer. Figure 3. Chronic papilledema with formation of optocilliary shunt vessels or collateral vessels. (Photo courtesy, Wayne Bixenman, MD).

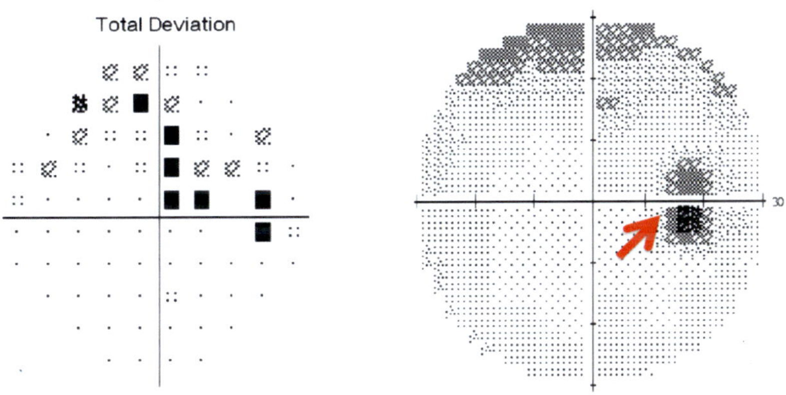

Figure 4. Right eye Humphrey Visual Field 30-2 grayscale map and associated total deviation map. Arrow points to increased physiologic blind spot.

Chronic central retinal venous obstruction from elevated ICP leads to dilation of preexisting venous channels on the disc's surface and the formation of optocilliary shunt vessels, also called collateral vessels (Figure 3).

There are no features of the disc appearance in papilledema to distinguish it from other causes of disc edema which are not associated with increased ICP, including optic neuritis and anterior ischemic optic neuropathy. Rather, there are clinical signs to suggest papilledema such as bilaterality (although this is not always the case and pronounced asymmetry or unilateral papilledema has been observed), preservation of central vision, and presence of associated symptoms such as headache, pulsatile tinnitus, and transient visual obscurations. [5]

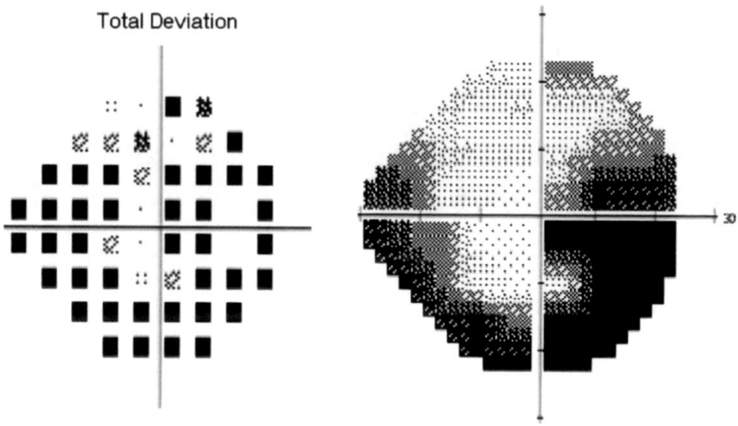

Figure 5. Right eye Humphrey Visual Field 24-2 grayscale map and associated total deviation map significant for arcuate visual field loss.

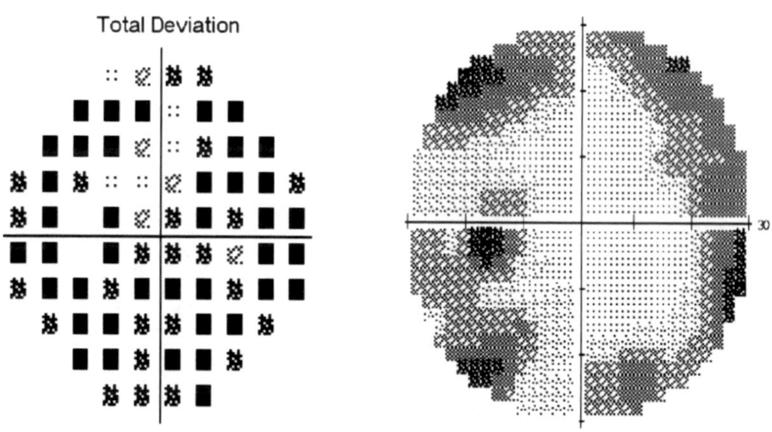

Figure 6. Left eye Humphrey Visual Field 30-2 grayscale map and associated total deviation map significant for general depression.

The main morbidity of papilledema is visual loss from axoplasmic flow stasis with resultant intraneuronal ischemia and permanent optic nerve damage. [6] In slow, chronic elevations of ICP, patients may present with visual changes such as an increase in the physiologic blind spot (Figure 4), arcuate visual field loss (Figure 5), generalized peripheral depression (Figure 6), and as a late sign, decreased central vision and even blindness. [6, 7]

The treatment for papilledema is to address the underlying causes of elevated ICP in an attempt to lower ICP through medical and/or surgical modalities. Specifically, in the setting of IIH, the mainstay of medical treatments includes weight loss and diuretics to decrease ICP. Even modest degrees of weight loss, 5-10 percent of total body weight, has been shown to improve clinical signs and symptoms of IIH. [8] In conjunction with weight loss, patients are frequently prescribed a diuretic, acetazolamide in particular, as a first line treatment to lower ICP. Acetazolamide is a carbonic anhydrase inhibitor that decreases the production of CSF and a dosage between 1 to 4 grams a day has been shown to be effective. [6] Second line agents include weaker carbonic anhydrase inhibitors, Furosemide and Topiramate.

Surgical treatments, such as optic nerve sheath fenestrations (ONSF) and neurosurgical shunt procedures, are required in fulminant cases or those refractory to maximal medical treatments with progression of vision loss. The specific surgical procedure undertaken depends on the patient's clinical picture and local resources available as both ONSF and neurosurgical shunt procedures are associated with potential complications. Patients with progressive visual deterioration in the absence of intolerable headaches may benefit from ONSF. In this procedure, a fistula between the subarachnoid space and orbital cavity is created by fenestration of the dural sheath surrounding the retrolaminar portion of the optic nerve, thus leading to a decrease in the pressure on the optic nerve. Because ONSF does not address the reduction of ICP itself, patients with predominant symptoms of headache in addition to progressive vision loss may require a CSF shunting procedure. [9]

In more recent years, transverse sinus stenting has also been performed as the majority of patients have been shown to exhibit non-thrombotic dural venous sinus stenosis of the transverse sinus on magnetic resonance venography. This collapse of the transverse sinus is thought to obstruct venous return and decrease CSF outflow and thus stents have been used to open portions of the transverse sinus. Several case series have shown that most patients who have undergone this procedure report significant improvement or resolution of their papilledema and symptoms. [10, 11]

Papilledema and Sleep-Disordered Breathing

The International Classification of Sleep Disorders, second edition (ICSD-2) subdivides sleep disorders into eight major categories: insomnia, sleep-related breathing disorders, hypersomnias of central origin, circadian rhythm disorders, parasomnias, and sleep-related movement disorders. [12] With increasing awareness during the past several decades, it is understood that sleep disorders may cause or worsen medical and psychiatric issues leading to poor occupational performance as well as cardiovascular and endocrine disorders. [13, 14] Their associations with ophthalmologic disorders have also been increasingly recognized and more specifically, there has been some evidence associating sleep-related breathing disorders to papilledema in particular.

Sleep-disordered breathing encompasses a spectrum of conditions sharing the common factor of losing a normal pattern of respiration during sleep. At the mild end of the spectrum are patients with only intermittent partial upper airway obstruction without serious disturbance of sleep, known as "simple snorers," and at the extreme end are those with the obesity-hypoventilation syndrome (OHS) or Pickwickian syndrome who demonstrate fragmented sleep in addition to day-time respiratory failure. [15] In between these extreme conditions exists obstructive sleep apnea (OSA), which is repetitive cessation of airflow during sleep due to collapse of the upper airway followed by hypoxemia until apnea is terminated by arousal and upper airway patency. [16] Approximately 90 percent of OHS patients have OSA. [15]

The first association between optic disc edema and OSA was reported by Bucci and Krohel [17] in 1988 regarding a case report of a patient whose disc edema resolved after surgical management of his OSA with a subsequent ICP measurement within normal limits of 170 mm H_2O. Since then, several cases have been reported in which patients with OSA and optic disc edema demonstrate both normal and elevated opening pressures on lumbar puncture with resolution or improvement of papilledema upon treatment for OSA. [18-21] Lee and colleagues [20] examined 6 cases of IIH in men with OSA, increased ICP, and bilateral optic disc swelling. All men had significant improvement or resolution of their papilledema after starting OSA treatment with continuous positive airway pressure (CPAP). Wolin and coauthors [22] reported a female with OSA, papilledema, and elevated ICP (500 mm H_2O) who was treated with biPAP, home oxygen therapy, acetazolamide, and weight reduction with dramatic improvement of papilledema over 2 months. In addition to patients with OSA, individuals further along the spectrum of sleep-disordered breathing with OHS have also been reported to exhibit elevated ICP and papilledema. [23, 24]

The association between OSA and increased ICP remains controversial. Purvin et al. [21] studied four patients with bilateral optic disc edema and OSA, who were all found to have normal daytime ICP measurements. However, continuous 24-hour ICP monitoring was also performed on one patient and demonstrated marked elevations of nocturnal ICP associated with apnea and arterial oxygen desaturation. The authors suggested that intermittent nocturnal elevations of ICP could produce papilledema. Sugita et al. [25] also reported a case series in which three patients with OSA and relatively normal daytime CSF pressures (mean, 260 mm H_2O) demonstrated transient and brief elevated nocturnal CSF pressure measurements during sleep with CSF pressure waves from 50 to 750 mm H_2O that was preceded or accompanied by an episode of apnea or hypopnea. They hypothesized that the elevated ICP occurs through various pathophysiological mechanisms, including transient hypoxia and hypercapnia during hypoventilation episodes causing the intracranial vascular volume to increase. In addition, the repetitive sympathetic activation during arousal from sleep may elevate systemic arterial pressure which results in increased intracranial perfusion pressure. [25, 26] The situation is further exacerbated during airway obstruction with increased intra-abdominal pressure and increased respiratory effort causing increased intrapleural pressure and leading to obstruction of cerebral venous drainage. [27, 28] Mojon and coauthors [29] also proposed that there is impaired optic nerve head blood flow autoregulation due to apneic episodes; failure of optic nerve autoregulation due to arterial hypertension and arteriosclerosis induced by OSA; prolonged hypoxic damage to the optic nerve; and imbalance between vasodilators and vasoconstrictors.

With progression of OSA, elevated ICP may persist and present similarly to IIH, thus explaining the presence of OSA and papilledema among those patients with both normal and elevated daytime ICP. Bruce et al. [30] reviewed 721 patients with IIH and found that 24 percent of men and 4 percent of women had co-existing OSA. In the study by Lee et al., [20] 6 out of 18 men with IIH had OSA. Despite the known association between IIH and OSA, the causality between OSA and IIH remains unclear. The question remains whether OSA is a comorbidity with obesity or if it is a cause of IIH that persists throughout the day. Waller and co-authors [7] suggest that if OSA is a cause of IIH, an explanation for this is that patients with OSA could develop enough intracranial hypertension during sleep to collapse the transverse sinuses, obstruct venous outflow, and cause continued elevated pressure during the day.

In a study conducted by Huseyinoglu et al., [31] OCT was used to measure the optic disc RNFL changes among mild, moderate, and severe OSA patients to investigate the progress of neurodegeneration. Although patients with optic disc edema were excluded from the study, there was a statistically significant reduction of peripapillary RNFL thickness in patients with severe OSA compared with the moderate group while there was an increase in the mild and moderate group compared with the control group. It was suggested that the optic nerve head passes through a stage of optic disc edema in the mild and moderate group with eventual secondary stage of reduction of RNFL thickness related to axonal loss in those with severe OSA. The authors recommended against the standard use of the OCT RNFL thickness measurement in OSA patients due to the confounding issues of both cerebral atrophy and disc edema. [31]

Despite the increasing recognition for the association between OSA and papilledema, the prevalence of optic nerve changes within the OSA population is not well known. To date, few prospective studies have evaluated this phenomena. In a study by Fraser et al., [32] fundus photographs were taken in patients undergoing overnight diagnostic polysomnography. Of the 215 patients, 59 percent had an apnea /hypopnea index (AHI) $\geq$ 15 events per hour (clinical diagnosis of OSA is AHI $\geq$ 5 with symptoms of snoring, daytime sleepiness, apneas, arousals or $\geq$ 15 without symptoms)[33] and 36 patients were diagnosed with severe OSA, although none of these individuals exhibited optic disc edema. In a separate study by Peter et al., [34] funduscopic examinations were performed on 35 patients with recently diagnosed OSA (within weeks) and visual symptoms suggestive of papilledema. None of the patients examined demonstrated papilledema and the authors concluded that papilledema is not a frequent finding in patients with OSA. [34] Of note, however, the patients in these prospective studies were all newly diagnosed with OSA and it is possible that papilledema may develop with time such as seen in cases of chronic OSA without treatment. More prospective studies with chronic OSA need to be conducted for better understanding. In the study by Purvin et al., [21] among the 4 patients with OSA and papilledema, 3 of the patients had been diagnosed with OSA for at least 1 year.

The association between sleep-disordered breathing and papilledema may be easily missed by clinicians in the setting of normal day-time ICP measurements. The incidence of visual loss in patients with IIH is 23 percent whereas 3 out of 4 patients in the study conducted by Purvin and colleagues [21] exhibited optic neuropathy. Although the patient group is small, the authors of the article suggest that OSA-related papilledema seem to be at higher risk for visual loss compared with patients with typical IIH. [21] Furthermore, when daytime ICP measurements are elevated, patients are more commonly diagnosed with IIH without determining if a sleep disorder component could be a contributing factor. Therefore, there should be a high index of suspicion for sleep-disordered breathing papilledema in patients with body habitus that predispose them to OSA, unexplained disc edema, and normal or elevated CSF pressures. Nocturnal measurements may be more useful in reaching a diagnosis but may be less clinically accessible.

Recognizing the association between OSA and papilledema (in the presence of normal neuroimaging results and normal CSF analysis) is vital for clinicians as treatment is available for OSA that may beneficially impact the progression of the patient's optic nerve disease. A prompt referral to a sleep specialist should be made for patients who present with symptoms suspicious for OSA so that the appropriate sleep study tests may be conducted for diagnosis.

Patients with OSA and disc edema in the setting of unremarkable neuroimaging results and CSF analysis and with normal or elevated daytime intracranial pressures should be treated for sleep apnea. Specifically, medical management with CPAP should be considered. Second line treatments include biPAP therapy or oral appliance devices. For patients with poorly tolerated or failed medical management, surgical management may be considered such as uvulopalatopharyngoplasty (most common procedure), genioglossus muscle advancement with hyoid myotomy, maxillomandibular advancement osteotomy, or tracheostomy for the severe, life-threatening presentations. [24] In addition, these patients should begin treatment with acetazolamide until papilledema symptoms resolve. For those patients whose disc edema fail to improve with these measures, it may be prudent to perform intracranial pressure monitoring prior to considering invasive forms of treatment such as optic nerve sheath fenestration or CSF shunting procedures. [35] More studies need to be conducted to better understand the pathophysiology and develop a standardized method of treatment.

Diseases of the optic nerve may have potentially devastating effects on patients. It is vital that primary care physicians, ophthalmologists, and sleep physicians work cooperatively and become aware of the association between sleep-related breathing disorder (in particular, OSA) and papilledema in an effort to reduce the morbidity and mortality of the disease process.

References

[1] Binder, DK, Horton, JC, Lawton, MT, McDermott, MW. Idiopathic intracranial hypertension *Neurosurgery*, 2004, 54(3), 538-51.

[2] Tso, MO, Hayreh, SS Optic disc edema in raised intracranial pressure IV. Axoplasmic transport in experimental papilledema *Arch Ophthalmol*, 1977, 95(8), 1458-62.

[3] Basic and clinical science course (BCSC) Section 5: Neuro-ophthalmology. In. San Francisco, CA: American Academy of Ophthalmology, 2013, 117.

[4] Scott, CJ, Kardon, RH, Lee, AG, et al. Diagnosis and grading of papilledema in patients with raised intracranial pressure using optical coherence tomography vs clinical expert assessment using a clinical staging scale. *Arch Ophthalmol*, 128(6), 705-11.

[5] Whiting, AS, Johnson, LN. Papilledema: clinical clues and differential diagnosis *Am Fam Physician*, 1992, 45(3), 1125-34.

[6] Lee, AG, Wall, M. Papilledema: are we any nearer to a consensus on pathogenesis and treatment? *Curr Neurol Neurosci Rep*,12(3), 334-9.

[7] Waller, EA, Bendel, RE, Kaplan, J. Sleep disorders and the eye. *Mayo Clin Proc*, 2008, 83(11), 1251-61.

[8] Kupersmith, MJ, Gamell, L, Turbin, R, et al. Effects of weight loss on the course of idiopathic intracranial hypertension in women. *Neurology*, 1998, 50(4), 1094-8.

[9] Jacobson, EE, Johnston, IH, McCluskey, P. The effect of optic nerve sheath decompression on CSF dynamics in pseudotumour cerebri and related conditions. *J Clin Neurosci*, 1999, 6(5), 375-7.

[10] Bussiere, M, Falero, R, Nicolle, D, et al. Unilateral transverse sinus stenting of patients with idiopathic intracranial hypertension *AJNR Am J Neuroradiol*, 31(4), 645-50.

[11] Ahmed, RM, Wilkinson, M, Parker, GD, et al. Transverse sinus stenting for idiopathic intracranial hypertension: a review of 52 patients and of model predictions. *AJNR Am J Neuroradiol*, 32(8), 1408-14.

[12] Sateia, M. ed. American Academy of Sleep Medicine, A. The international classification of sleep disorders, 2nd ed. Vol. Diagnostic and coding manual. Westchester, IL: American Academy of Sleep Medicine, 2005, 1-297.

[13] Lockley, SW, Barger, LK, Ayas, NT, et al. Effects of health care provider work hours and sleep deprivation on safety and performance. *Jt Comm J Qual Patient Saf*, 2007, 33(11 Suppl), 7-18.
[14] Copinschi, G. Metabolic and endocrine effects of sleep deprivation *Essent Psychopharmacol*, 2005, 6(6), 341-7.
[15] Grunstein, RR, Wilcox, I., Sleep-disordered breathing and obesity *Baillieres Clin Endocrinol Metab*, 1994, 8(3), 601-28.
[16] Sullivan, CE, Issa, FG, Berthon-Jones, M, Saunders, NA. Pathophysiology of sleep apnea In: Saunders NA, Sullivan CE, eds. Sleep and Breathing. New York: Marcel Dekker, 1984.
[17] Bucci, FA, Jr., Krohel, GB. Optic nerve swelling secondary to the obstructive sleep apnea syndrome *Am J Ophthalmol*, 1988, 105(4), 428-30.
[18] Hett, KL, Chutter, LJ, Hassan, M, Okosieme, OE. Declining vision: saved by a tracheostomy *BMJ Case Rep*, 2013.
[19] Javaheri, S, Qureshi, Z, Golnik, K. Resolution of papilledema associated with OSA treatment *J Clin Sleep Med*, 7(4), 399-400.
[20] Lee, AG, Golnik, K, Kardon, R, et al. Sleep apnea and intracranial hypertension in men. *Ophthalmology*, 2002, 109(3), 482-5.
[21] Purvin, VA, Kawasaki, A, Yee, RD. Papilledema and obstructive sleep apnea syndrome *Arch Ophthalmol*, 2000, 118(12), 1626-30.
[22] Wolin, MJ, Brannon, WL. Disk edema in an overweight woman. *Surv Ophthalmol*, 1995, 39(4), 307-14.
[23] Meyer, JS, Gotham, J, Tazaki, Y, Gotoh, F. Cardiorespiratory syndrome of extreme obesity with papilledema Report of a fatal case with electroencephologographic, metabolic, and necropsy studies. *Neurology*, 1961, 11, 950-8.
[24] Grover, DP. Obstructive sleep apnea and ocular disorders. *Curr Opin Ophthalmol*, 21(6), 454-8.
[25] Sugita, Y, Iijima, S, Teshima, Y, et al. Marked episodic elevation of cerebrospinal fluid pressure during nocturnal sleep in patients with sleep apnea hypersomnia syndrome *Electroencephalogr Clin Neurophysiol*, 1985, 60(3), 214-9.
[26] Eisensehr, I, Ehrenberg, BL, Noachtar, S, et al. Platelet activation, epinephrine, and blood pressure in obstructive sleep apnea syndrome *Neurology*, 1998, 51(1), 188-95.
[27] McNamara, ME. Idiopathic intracranial hypertension without papilledema: related to sleep apnea? *Arch Neurol*, 1992, 49(1), 14.

[28] Rich, GB. Article reviewed: Papilledema and obstructive sleep apnea syndrome *Sleep Med*, 2001, 2(3), 259-61.

[29] Mojon, DS, Mathis, J, Zulauf, M, et al. Optic neuropathy associated with sleep apnea syndrome *Ophthalmology*, 1998, 105(5), 874-7.

[30] Bruce, BB, Kedar, S, Van, Stavern, GP, et al. Idiopathic intracranial hypertension in men. *Neurology*, 2009, 72(4), 304-9.

[31] Huseyinoglu, N, Ekinci, M, Ozben, S, et al. Optic disc and retinal nerve fiber layer parameters as indicators of neurodegenerative brain changes in patients with obstructive sleep apnea syndrome *Sleep Breath*, 18(1), 95-102.

[32] Fraser, CL, Bliwise, DL, Newman, NJ, et al. A prospective photographic study of the ocular fundus in obstructive sleep apnea *J Neuroophthalmol*, 33(3), 241-6.

[33] Epstein, LJ, Kristo, D, Strollo, PJ, Jr. et al. Clinical guideline for the evaluation, management and long-term care of obstructive sleep apnea in adults *J Clin Sleep Med*, 2009, 5(3), 263-76.

[34] Peter, L, Jacob, M, Krolak-Salmon, P, et al. Prevalence of papilloedema in patients with sleep apnoea syndrome: a prospective study. *J Sleep Res*, 2007, 16(3), 313-8.

[35] Lee, AG. Three questions on the role of sleep apnea syndrome in optic disc edema *Arch Ophthalmol*, 2001, 119(8), 1225.

In: Eye Diseases ...
Editor: Mingwu Wang

ISBN: 978-1-63482-894-9

Chapter 10

Nonarteritic Anterior Ischemic Optic Neuropathy and Obstructive Sleep Apnea

Todd W. Altenbernd*, MD and Whitney A. Smith, MD
Department of Ophthalmology and Vision Science,
University of Arizona College of Medicine, AZ, US

Case Presentation

A 65 year-old man with a history of hypertension and borderline diabetes awakens one morning with painless blurry vision, a perception of muted colors and dimness of light in the left eye. He reports no additional neurological or cardiovascular symptoms. On examination the affected eye has a moderate decrease in visual acuity, color perception, and a Marcus-Gunn pupil. Dilated examination is normal for age with the exception of edema and a few splinter hemorrhages in the lower half of the left optic nerve head (Figure 1). Formal visual field testing reveals a moderate, diffuse decrease in sensitivity and a more pronounced depression of the upper half of the visual field in the left eye (Figure 2). The visual field of the right eye is normal. Neurological examination shows cranial nerves 3-12 are intact bilaterally with no evidence

*Email: taltenbernd@eyes.arizona.edu

of focal deficits. The patient denies jaw claudication, temporal headaches, unexplained weight loss, fever, chills, night sweats and shoulder or back pain. A Westergren erythrocyte sedimentation rate (ESR) and C reactive protein (CRP) are both normal.

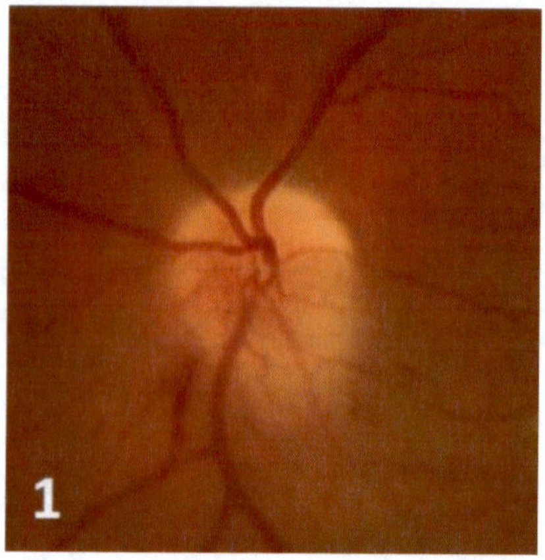

Figure 1. Color fundus photograph of nonarteritic anterior ischemic optic neuropathy, left eye. The superior nerve shows pallor after prior edema has resolved. The inferior half of the disc remains edematous with dilated vessels nasally and splinter hemorrhages just below the disc.

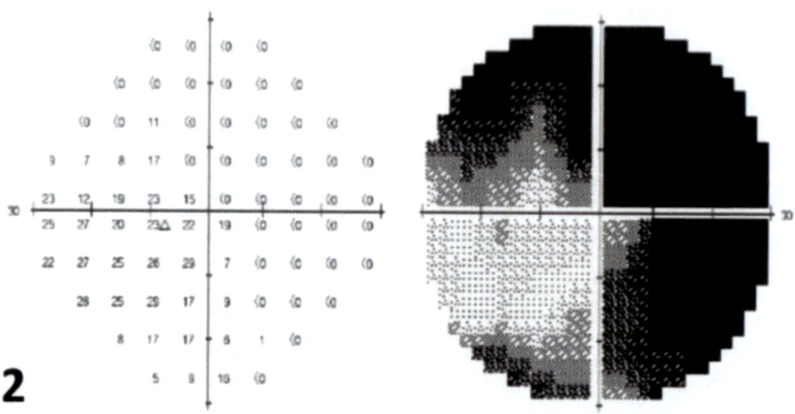

Figure 2. Visual field of the same left eye after nonarteritic anterior ischemic optic neuropathy. Left eye Humphrey 30-2 visual field shows a dense superior incomplete hemifield depression and a dense inferior nasal depression. The fellow eye showed a normal visual field.

Nonarteritic Anterior Ischemic Optic Neuropathy: An Overview

Nonarteritic anterior ischemic optic neuropathy (NAION) is the most common form of non-glaucomatous optic neuropathy in adults over 50 years of age. It may result in permanently decreased visual acuity and a variety of visual field deficits. Patients often report a combination of painlessly decreased visual acuity, visual field constriction or defects, muted color perception and a relative dimness of light seen by the affected eye.

In 73% of cases visual acuity loss is first noticed upon awakening. [1] Visual acuity may vary widely from normal to no light perception. The distribution of acuities varies with one study finding 67% of all NAION eyes to have an initial visual acuity of 20/60 or better, [2] but another reported only 25% to be in this range. [3] All patients demonstrate visual field deficits with the most common abnormalities being superior or inferior incomplete altitudinal defects (Figure 2). Another constant finding is the presence of a relative afferent pupillary defect, also called a Marcus-Gunn pupil, which is present unless there is optic nerve disease in both eyes and the damage is symmetric. Here the affected eye constricts less briskly or may dilate when a bright light is swung from the unaffected eye to the affected eye. This test indicates compromised signal transmission of one optic nerve compared to the other and is relatively unaffected by cataracts, corneal opacities or vitreous opacities. Finally, in NAION, fundoscopic examinations during the first few weeks show focal altitudinal or diffuse edema of the optic nerve with splinter hemorrhages frequently present on the nerve (Figure 1). [4]

Arteritic anterior ischemic optic neuropathy (AAION) is a less common optic neuropathy that presents very similarly to NAION. AAION must be ruled out to make the diagnosis of NAION. This is usually done through a combination of history, physical examination, laboratory testing and sometimes a biopsy of the temporal artery. The vast majority of cases of AAION result from temporal arteritis (also called giant cell arteritis), which is a systemic inflammatory disease of medium and large-sized arteries. Typically AAION patients report a variety of additional symptoms including jaw claudication, temporal headaches and tenderness, unexplained weight loss, polymyalgia rheumatica-type symptoms, fever, chills and night sweats. On examination they may have tenderness in the temporal region with skin redness and an underlying nodule. The temporal arteries may be pulseless. An elevated ESR and CRP are highly suggestive of AAION and immediate high dose systemic steroid treatment is indicated to reduce the risk of blindness in the fellow eye as well as the likelihood of cardiovascular and cerebrovascular occlusions.

The natural history of NAION can include improvement or worsening of visual acuity and visual fields during the first 6 months post event. [2, 3] In those with initial vision of 20/70 or better, visual acuity at 24 months improved by 3 lines or more in 31-36% and worsened by 3 lines or more in 18-22%. [2, 3] The occurrence of an NAION in the fellow eye is 14.7-26% over 5 years. [3, 5] This is considerably greater than a second NAION in the same eye, which has been reported to occur in only 3-5% patients over 5 years. [6] There is evidence to suggest that systemic risk factors for occurrence in the second eye may exist, particularly diabetes mellitus and a visual acuity worse than 20/200 in the first eye. [3]

After the ischemic insult, the optic nerve undergoes sequential changes in a predictable pattern in NAION. Optic disc edema is present on fundoscopic examination, with localized splinter hemorrhages often noted on the disc. Edema may initially be localized to the superior or inferior disc but may later be seen to involve the entire disc. This edema typically resolves in 4-8 weeks and is replaced by nerve head pallor. Pallor may be seen as early as 2-3 weeks and may become more prominent as the edema resolves. Visual field defects commonly correspond to the area of optic nerve edema. [7]

The reported incidence of NAION varies widely from 2.3-82 in 100,000 and it affects men and women equally. [9-12] This large range in values likely reflects the differences in methods and populations investigated. The best estimates in the United States are 50 per 100,000 in those over age 40 and 82 in 100,000 for those over age 68.

Risk factors for NAION are multiple and show great variation among studies. The highest risk of NAION occurs in an eye undergoing cataract surgery whose fellow eye had experienced a prior NAION. The relative risk increases 3.6-7.4 fold in this situation with the rate of NAION initially increasing over the first several months after cataract surgery and then approaching the pre-cataract rate thereafter. The median time to NAION after cataract extraction was 2.8 months. [5] The most consistently reported systemic association of NAION is with diabetes mellitus, but hypertension, ischemic heart disease, thyroid disease, COPD and atherosclerosis have all been found to occur in a higher proportion in patients with NAION than the general population. Additionally, NAION occurs more frequently in Caucasians and in those over 50 years of age. [10, 13] Another consistent finding is a cup to disc ratio of less than 0.3 and a small optic nerve. [14-18]

Several medications have also been linked to NAION. Amiodarone can produce a clinical picture similar to NAION but the onset of symptoms is insidious and the optic nerve edema is bilateral. Here the optic neuropathy improves with cessation of the medication but the optic nerve edema takes longer to resolve than with a typical NAION. [19, 20] Sildenafil, tadalafil and vardenafil are erectile dysfunction (ED) medications (phosphodiesterase-5 inhibitors) that are associated with the ocular side effects of a bluish hue, blurry vision, increased light sensitivity and color vision abnormalities. These side effects are uncommon, dose-dependent and reversible. There have been implications that these medications induce NAION and a number of the reported cases have been temporally related to ED medication dosing. [21, 22] However, with over 50 million prescriptions written for a group that is generally at higher risk for NAION it is difficult to assume a causal relationship. It may, however, be of value to counsel patients with a cup to disc ratio of less than 0.3 who are considering phospodiesterase-5 inhibitor use about the possible increased risk of NAION. [6]

There are several hypotheses regarding the cause of tissue damage in NAION but the true mechanism is not precisely known. All theories share the underlying concept of vascular insufficiency to the optic nerve from hypoperfusion [13] or vascular occlusion. [23] Reports addressing the possibility of intermittent hypoperfusion have been conflicting and theories of autoregulation abnormalities at the level of the posterior ciliary arteries are difficult to investigate. While histopathological changes consistent with infarction are frequently seen behind the lamina of the optic nerve in NAION there have been little or no findings of vascular occlusion in this location. [24] In contrast, vascular occlusion of the posterior ciliary arteries is commonly seen during histopathology evaluation of AAION.

Additionally, an intrascleral compartment syndrome has been proposed stemming from the combination of optic disc edema, a small cup and limited area for expansion of the optic disc at the level of the scleral ring. Most of the attempted treatments have tried to limit this positive feedback cycle of edema, expansion, axonal damage and more edema. A final theory, which explains the visual recovery seen in NAION, suggests that subretinal fluid is present at the time of incident but is subsequently resorbed over time. This has been demonstrated in a number of acute NAION patients by ocular coherence tomography (OCT). [5]

Currently there are no class I studies to support the prevention of or efficacious treatment for NAION. Optic nerve decompression has been the most rigorously tested treatment for this disease with a multicenter randomized controlled clinical trial conducted in the United States. This modality attempts to decompress the proposed compartment syndrome of the edematous optic nerve by decreasing the cerebral spinal fluid pressure around the optic nerve sheath. This is achieved by fenestrating the intraorbital optic nerve sheath in a region a few centimeters posterior to its connection to the globe. However, the study was stopped after 24 months with no benefits attributed to optic nerve sheath decompression over observation alone. [26, 27]

Transvitreal Neurotomy is another approach to decompress the optic nerve. Here a surgical blade is used to cut the scleral ring surrounding the optic disc. This incision is made from within the eye and in theory allows the edematous nerve to expand, reducing the damage caused by a localized compartment syndrome. A small case series suggested improvement relative to historical controls as 5 of 7 eyes improved significantly. However, there have been no follow-up studies to date. [28]

Hyperbaric oxygen treatment has also been studied. The theory here is that increased oxygen delivery to the compromised optic nerve may save axons, but there has been no evidence of improvement over historical controls in small case series. [29] Systemic steroids have similarly been proposed to reduce optic nerve edema and thus limit the compartment syndrome surrounding the nerve. A large pseudorandomized trial where patients self-selected treatment with short term high dose systemic steroids versus observation showed a significant benefit in preserving visual acuity and visual field in the steroid group. [2] To the contrary, smaller case series paired against historical controls not only failed to show a benefit from similar steroid regimens, they also observed a number of steroid related side effects. [30, 31] Currently, there is no preponderance of evidence to support the benefit of using systemic steroids in the treatment of NAION.

Intravitreal triamcinolone injections showed some promise in a small case series as compared to historical controls. [32] Although there were no systemic side effects, historically this route of triamcinolone administration has a relatively high rate of eye pressure elevation, which can increase the potential for glaucoma formation in the treated eye. Intravitreal anti-VEGF antibodies such as bevacizumab and ranibizumab have been shown to decrease vascular permeability in a number of ocular diseases. Therefore, they theoretically could decrease vascular permeability at the level of the optic nerve without many of the complications inherent in intravitreal steroid injections. In a small pseudorandomized study 17 patients chose a single injection of bevacizumab (Avastin) while 8 chose careful follow-up. There was no difference in vision or visual field between groups. [33] In another case series of 17 eyes a single injection of ranibizumab (Lucentis) was compared to historical controls and found to have a beneficial effect on visual acuity. [34] The discrepancy between these two studies may stem from differences in the severity of optic nerve damage. In the first study, [33] visual acuity was significantly better initially after the NAION and historically these eyes do not improve as much as the eyes that began with more substantial damage. [2] Additionally, although bevacizumab and ranibizumab work similarly in a variety of eye diseases at the standard quantities used, here it is possible that ranibizumab may be superior for NAION. The remarkable response to ranibizumab as compared to historical controls warrants further investigation.

Aspirin has been studied as a potential treatment for acute NAION. In a retrospective review of aspirin use before and during the course of an NAION there was no evidence to suggest a beneficial effect on visual acuity or visual fields. [35] Alternatively, the role of aspirin as a preventative tool is less clear. A review of the Optic Neuropathy Decompression Trial data and a retrospective review of 118 NAION cases suggested no beneficial effects of aspirin in reducing the rate of NAION in the fellow eye. [3, 36] In contrast, another large retrospective study suggested a protective effect over the first 2 years but no statistically significant effect by 5 years. [37] Finally, a retrospective study of 100 patients showed a large and statistically significant benefit at preventing an NAION in the fellow eye. [38] However, aspirin is not routinely recommended at present by ophthalmologists during or following an occurrence of NAION.

Brimonidine tartrate is a topical alpha 2 agonist that has demonstrated neuroprotective effects in rats and monkeys subjected to traumatic optic neuropathy and glaucoma, respectively. Two small studies with human subjects failed to show a beneficial effect of brimonidine tartrate on acute NAION. [39, 40] Transcorneal electrostimulation is a novel treatment strategy. In a case series of 3 eyes, one eye showed a significant improvement in visual acuity. Unlike other studies where treatment began 2 weeks or less from the onset of NAION, this study included eyes that were 4-24 months post event. [41] Since NAION natural history studies have shown no significant changes in visual acuity or visual fields beyond 6 months post event this effect of neurostimulation is difficult to explain. [2] In view of a single, very small study any conclusions regarding efficacy are guarded.

Nonarteritic Anterior Ischemic Optic Neuropathy and Obstructive Sleep Apnea

Since in the majority of NAION cases, patients discovered visual loss upon first awakening or at first opportunity to use vision critically after sleeping, [1] the association between the development of NAION and sleep conditions become an interest of investigation. To date, five studies linking obstructive sleep apnea (OSA) to NAION were identified in a literature search (Table 1). [43-46] Four of these were case-control studies with matched controls. [42, 43, 45, 46] A fifth study was a case series comparing patients to historical controls from a large population-based study performed at other facilities. [44] Notably, there was a limited quantity of literature and a wide variety of diagnostic criteria used to define OSA.

In summary, there appears to be sufficient evidence to support an independent association between OSA and NAION. The differences between the 5 studies with respect to the prevalence of known OSA risk factors, criteria for diagnosis and evaluation methods make it difficult to compare or combine any 2 studies. However, in the studies by the groups of Biligin and Mojon, the controls were well matched in all known OSA risk factors and the calculated odds ratios convey a clinically and statistically significant association with NAION. [43, 45] Further support of such an independent association comes from another study, which used historical controls from a separate, independent, population-based study. [44] Although the proportion of known OSA risk factors was not well matched in this study, the method of a stratified univariate comparison across several risk factors showed a large and statistically significant result for all factors considered. [44] Lesser support stems from the study by Arda, et al., which shows a trend without statistical significance at the 95% confidence level. [42] Here the controls were well matched in all but neck circumference. Any adjustments for neck circumference would be small and would further reduce the association between the mild-severe OSA and NAION. Finally, the study by Li, et al. was unique in that the gold standard of polysomnography was not used to determine OSA and thus resulted in reduced strength of the findings. [46] The sleep apnea scale of the sleep disorders questionnaire (SA-SDQ) used in this study has the benefit of being non-invasive, inexpensive and easily administered compared to polysomnography, and the results suggested that OSA was indeed associated with NAION.

Table 1. Summary of NAION-OSA studies

First author	Criteria	Odds Ratio	95% CI Low	95% CI High		Comments
Arda [42]	AHI>5 mild-severe	3.1	0.60	16	p>0.05	20 NAION, 20 matched controls underwent polysomnography. AHI >5 was the criterion for OSA. OSA was seen at a much higher prevalence in NAION (85%) and controls (65%) than in the general population (29%).
Biligin [43]	AHI>19 moderate-severe	4.4	1.3	15	p<0.05	27 NAION, 27 matched controls underwent polysomnography. AHI >=20 was the criterion for SAS.
Palombi [44]	AHI>15 moderate-severe	36.4	10.3	129	p<0.001	20 consecutive NAION patients underwent polysomnography and were compared to a large multicenter study which used the same criterion of AHI>15. Both NAION and control groups were stratified into quartiles for known risk factors and univariate analysis was performed on each factor.
Mojon [45]	RDI>10 mild-severe	11.2	1.95	64.4	p<0.005	17 NAION and 17 controls underwent polysomnography. RDI was used instead of AHI in this study and a value >10 was set as the threshold.
Li [46]	SA-SDQ >36 for men >32 for women Unknown severity	2.62	1.03	6.60	P<0.05	73 NAION and 73 matched controls were assessed for SAS using the SA-SDQ but no polysomnography was utilized.

OSA: Obstructive sleep apnea
AHI: Apnea hypopnea index
NAION: Nonarteritic ischemic optic neuropathy
RDI: Respiratory disturbance index
SA-SDQ: Sleep apnea scale of the sleep disorders questionnaire

A commonly shared pathophysiology of NAION is vascular insufficiency to the optic nerve from hypoperfusion. [13] Hence several mechanisms have been proposed to explain the link between NAION and OSA. The cascade of events during OSA such as hypoxia, hypercapnia, sympathetic activation and arterial hypertension, may alter optic nerve head blood supply by affecting arterial autoregulation. Additionally, episodic hypoperfusion can theoretically lead to nitric oxide and endothelin imbalance, which can also affect blood flow to the nerve. It is also possible that prolonged hypoxic episodes and increased intracranial pressure during OSA may cause direct damage to the optic nerve itself. [23, 45, 51, 52]

Continuous positive airway pressure (CPAP) devices are commonly used as an effective treatment of OSA. To date, two studies investigated the association of CPAP treatment for OSA and the development of NAION. [11, 53] One study reviewed 108 cases of NAION diagnosed over a one-year period by the neuro-ophthalmology department at Wills Eye Hospital in Philadelphia. [53] A chart review identified 4 eyes of 3 patients who developed an NAION while receiving CPAP for OSA. The diagnosis of OSA was confirmed by the patient's pulmonologist and the duration of CPAP use ranged from 4 months to 6 years. One of these patients experienced sequential bilateral NAIONs while being treated with CPAP. This review study indicated that CPAP therapy does not eliminate the risks for NAION in patients with OSA, but the systemic efficacy and level of compliance with CPAP treatment were not reported. On the other hand, NAION occurs without OSA and thus non-OSA factors may have played a role.

The other study reviewed diagnostic and procedure codes from over 2 million individuals enrolled within a single healthcare plan over a 7-year interval. [11] A multivariate analysis showed that individuals with untreated OSA were statistically more likely to develop an NAION compared to those without OSA.

Similarly, when OSA patients treated with CPAP were compared to individuals without OSA the multivariate analysis showed a trend toward an increased risk for NAION but this did not reach statistical significance. [11] Overall, it appears that NAION may still occur in OSA even when treated by CPAP although there is some evidence to suggest that CPAP may provide a protective effect.

References

[1] Hayreh SS, Podhajsky PA, Zimmerman B. Nonarteritic anterior ischemic optic neuropathy: time of onset of visual loss. *Am. J. Ophthalmol.* 1997 Nov;124(5):641-7.

[2] Hayreh S, Zimmerman B. Nonarteritic Anterior Ischemic Optic Neuropathy: Natural History of Visual Outcome. *Ophthalmology. 2008:115(2): 298-305.*

[3] Newman NJ, Schere R, Langenberg P, et al.: Ischemic Optic Neuropathy Decompression Trial Research Group: The fellow eye in NAION: report from the Ischemic Optic Neuropathy Decompression Trial follow-up study. *Am. J. Ophthalmol* 2002, 134(3):317-328.

[4] Arnold AC, Hepler RS. Natural history of nonarteritic anterior ischemic optic neuropathy *J. Neuroophthalmol.* 1994 Jun;14(2):66-9.

[5] Lam BL, Jabaly-Habib H, Al-Sheikh N, Pezda M, Guirgis MF, Feuer WJ, McCulley TJ.: Risk of non-arteritic anterior ischaemic optic neuropathy (NAION) after cataract extraction in the fellow eye of patients with prior unilateral NAION. *Br. J. Ophthalmol.* 2007;91:585-587.

[6] Miller, Neil. Pathogensis and Management of Nonarteritic Anterior Ischemic Optic Neuropathy. *J. Neuro-Ophthalmol* 2011; 31:21-e3.

[7] Chen T, Song D, Shan G, Wang K, Wang Y et al. (2013) The Association between Diabetes Mellitus and Nonarteric Anterior Ischemic Optic Neuropathy: A Systemic Review and Meta-Analysis *PLoS ONE* 8(9) e76653.

[8] Hayreh S. Ischemic optic neuropathy. Progress in Retinal and Eye Research 28 (2009) 34-62.

[9] Hattenhauer MG, Leavitt JA, Hodge DO, Grill R, Gray D. Incidence of Nonarteritic Anterior Ischemic Optic Neuropathy. *Am. J. Ophthalmol.* 1997 123(1):103-7.

[10] Lee M, Grossman D, Arnold A, Sloan F. Incidence of nonarteritic ischemic optic neuropathy: increased risk among diabetic patients. *Ophthalmology*. 2011 May; 118(5): 959-963.

[11] Stein J, Kim D, Mundy K, Talwar N, Nan B, Chervin R, Musch D. The Association Between Glaucomatous and Other Causes of Optic Neuropathy and Sleep Apnea. *Am. J. Ophthalmol.* 2011 December; 152(6):989-998.

[12] Johnson L, Arnold A. Incidence of Nonarteritic and Ateritic Anterior Ischemic Optic Neuropathy Population-Based Study in the State of Missouri and Los Angeles County, California. *Journal of Neuro-ophthalmology* 14(1);18-44 1994.

[13] Hayreh SS, Zimmerman MB, Podhajsky P, Alward WL. Nocturnal arterial hypotension and its role in optic nerve head and ocular ischemic disorders. *Am. J. Ophthalmol.* 1994 May 15;117(5):603-24.

[14] Beck RW, Savino PJ, Repka MX, Schatz NJ, Serfot RC. Optic disc structure in anterior ischemic optic neuropathy. *Ophthalmology* 1984 Nov;91(11):1334-7.

[15] Beck RW, Servais GE, Hayreh SS Anterior ischemic optic neuropathy IX. Cup-to-disc ratio and its role in pathogenesis. *Ophthalmology* 1987 Nov;94(11):1503-8.

[16] Doro S, Lessell S. Cup-disc ratio and ischemic optic neuropathy. *Arch. Ophthalmol.* 1985 Aug;103(8):1143-4.

[17] Feit RH, Tomsak RL, Ellenberger C. Structural factors in the pathogenesis of ischemic optic neuropathy. *Am. J. Ophthalmol.* 1984 Jul 15;998(1):105-8.

[18] Mansour AM, Shoch D, Logani S. Optic disc size in ischemic optic neuropathy. *Am. J. Ophthalmol.* 1988 15;106(5):587-9.

[19] Li J, Tripathi RC, Tripathi BJ. Drug-Induced Ocular Disorders. *Drug Safety.* 2008; 31(2) 127-141.

[20] Murphy M, Murphy J. Amiodarone and optic neuropathy: the heart of the matter. *J. Neuroophthalmol.* 2005;25:232-236.

[21] Pomeranz H, Bhavar A. Nonarteritic ischemic optic neuropathy developing soon after use of sidenafil (viagra) a report of seven new cases. *J. Neurophthalmol.* 2005;25:9-13.

[22] Cunningham A, Smith K. Anterior ischemic optic neuropathy associated with viagra. *J. Neuroophthalmol.* 2001;21:22-25.

[23] Arnold AC, Pathogenesis of Nonarteritic Anterior Ischemic Optic Neuropathy. *J. Neuro-Ophthalmol.* 2003;23: 157-163.

[24] Knox DL, Kerrison JB, Green WR. Histopathologic studies of ischemic optic neuropathy. Tr. Am. Ophth. Soc. 2000;98:203-22.

[25] Hedges TR, Vuong LN, Gonzalez-Garcia AO, Mendoza-Santiesteban CE, Amaro-Quierza ML. Subretinal fluid from anterior ischemic optic neuropathy demonstrated by optical coherence tomography. *Arch. Ophthalmol.* 2008 Jun;126(6):812-5.

[26] Dickersin K, Manheimer E, Li T. Surgery for nonarteritic anterior ischemic optic neuropathy. *The Cochrane Library* 2013 issue 5;1-19.

[27] Ischemic Optic Neuropathy Decompression Trial Research Group. Ischemic Optic Neuropathy Decompression Trial: Twenty-Four-Month Update. *Arch. Opthalmol.* 2000;118:793-798.

[28] Soheilian M, Kochek A, Yazdani S, Payman GA. Transvitreal optic neurotomy for nonarteritic anterior ischemic optic neuropathy. *Retina* 2003;23(5):692-7.

[29] Arnold AC, Hepler RS, Lieber M, Alexander JM. Hyperbaric oxygen therapy for nonarteritic anterior ischemic optic neuropathy. *Am. J. Ophthalmol.* 1996 Oct;122(4):535-41.

[30] Rebolleda G, Perez-Lopez M, Casas-Llera P, Contreras I, Munoz-Negrete FJ. Visual and anatomical outcomes of non-arteritic anterior ischemic optic neuropathy with high-dose systemic corticosteroids. *Graefes Arch. Clin. Exp. Ophthalmol.* 2013(251):255-260.

[31] Kinori K, Ben-Bassat I, Wasserzug Y, Chetrit A, Huna-Baron R. Visual outcome of mega-dose intravenous corticosteroid treatement in non-arteritic anterior ischemic optic neuropathy – retrospective analysis. *BMC Ophthalmology* 2014, 14:62.

[32] Radoi C, Garcia T, Brugniart C, Ducasse A, Arndt C: Intravitreal triamcinolone injection in non-arteritic anterior ischemic optic neuropathy. *Graefes Arch. Clin. Exp. Ophthalmol.* 2014, 252:339-345.

[33] Rootman DB, Gill HS, Margolin EA. Intravitreal bevacizumab for the treatment of nonarteritic Ischemic optic neuropathy: a prospective trial. *Eye* 2013 (27)538-544.

[34] Saatci AO, Taskin O, Selver OB, Yaman A, Bajin MS. Efficacy of Intravitreal Ranibizumab Injection in Acute Nonarteritic Ischemic Optic Neuropathy: A Long-Term Follow Up. *The Open Ophthalmology Journal* 2013 (7)58-62.

[35] Botelho PJ, Johnson LN, Arnold AC. The Effect of Aspirin on the Visual Outcome of Nonarteritic Anterior Ischemic Optic Neuropathy. *Am. J. Ophthalmol.* 1996 121(4)450-451.

[36] Salomon O, Huna-Baron R, Steinberg DM, et al. Role of aspirin in reducing the frequency of second eye involvement in patients with non-arteritic anterior ischaemic optic neuropathy. *Eye* 1999, 13(Pt 3a):357-359.

[37] Beck RW, Hayreh SS, Podhajky PA, et al. Asprin therapy in nonarteritic anterior ischemic optic neuropathy. *Am. J. Ophthalmol.* 1997, 123(2):193-198.

[38] Kupersmith MJ, Frohman L, Sanderson M, et al.: Aspirin reduces the incidence of second eye NAION: a retrospective study. *J. Neuroophthalmol.* 1997, 17(4):250-253.

[39] Fazzone HE, Kupersmith MJ, Leibman J. Does topical Brimonidine tartarate help NAION? *Br. J. Ophthalmol.* 2003 1193-1194.

[40] Wihelm B, Ludtke H, Wilhelm H, BRAION study group. Efficacy and tolerability of 0.2% brimonidine tartrate for the treatment of acute non-arteritic anterior ischemic optic neuropathy (NAION): a 3-month, double-masked, randomized, placebo-controlled trial. *Graefe's Arch. Clin. Exp. Ophthalmol.* (2006) 244:551-558.

[41] Jujikado T, Morimoto T, Matsushita K, Shimojo H, Okasw Y, Tano Y. Effect of Transcorneal Electrical Stimulation in Patients with Nonarteritic Ischemic Optic Neuropathy or Traumatic Optic Neuropathy. *Jpn. J. Ophthalmol.* 2006;50:266-273.

[42] Arda H, Birer S, Aksu M, Ismailogullari S, et al. Obstructive Sleep apnoea prevalence in non-arteritic anterior ischaemic optic neuropathy. *Br. J. Ophthalmol.* 2013;97:206-209.

[43] Bilgin G, Koban Y, Arnold A. Nonarteritic Anterior Ischemic Optic Neuropathy and Obstructive Sleep Apnea. *Journal of Neuro-Ophthalmology* 2013;33:232-234.

[44] Palombi K, Renard E, Levy P, Chiquet C, Deschaux Ch, Romanet JP, Pepin JL. Non-arteritic anterior ischaemic optic neuropathy is nearly systematically associated with obstructive sleep apnoea. *Br. J. Ophthalmol.* 2006;90:879-882.

[45] Mojon D, Hedges T, Ehrenberg B, Karam E, Goldblum D, Abou-Chebl A, Gugger M, Mathis J. Association Between Sleep Apnea Syndrome and Nonarteritic Anterior Ischemic Optic Neuropathy. *Arch. Ophthalmol.* 2002;120:601-605.

[46] Li J, McGwin G, Baphiades MS, Owsley C. Non-arteritic anterior ischaemic optic neuropathy and presumed sleep apnoea syndrome screened by the Sleep Apnea scale of the Sleep Disorder Questionnaire (SA-SDQ). *Br. J. Ophthalmol.* 2007;91:1524-1527.

[47] Young T, Eyal Shahar, F. Javier Nieto, Susan Redline, Anne B.Newman, Daniel J. Gottlieb, Joyce A. Walsleben, Laurel Finn, Paul Enright, Jonathan M. Samet, the Sleep Heart Health Study Research Group. Predictors of Sleep-Disordered Breathing in Community-Dwelling Adults: The Sleep Heart Health Study. *Arch. Intern.* Med. 2002;162(8):893-900.

[48] Douglas AB, Bornstein R, Nino-Murcia G, Keenan S, Miles L, Zarcone V, Guilleminault C, Dement W. The Sleep Disorders Questionnaire I: Creation and Multivariate Structure of SDQ. *Sleep* 17(2) 160-167.

[49] Weatherwax KJ, Lin X, Marzec ML, Malow BA. Obstructive Sleep Apnea in epilepsy patients: the Sleep Apnea scale of the Sleep Disorders Questionnaire (SA-SDQ) is a useful screening instrument for obstructive sleep apnea in a disease-specific population. *Sleep Med.* 2003 Nov;4(6):517-21.

[50] Economou NT, Dikeos D, Andrews N, Foldvary-Schaefer N. Use of Sleep Apnea Scale of the Sleep Disorder Questionnaire (SA-SDQ) in adults with epilepsy. *Epilepsy & Behavior*. 2014 31:123-126.

[51] Mojon D, Mathis J, Zulauf M. Optic neuropathy associated with sleep apnea syndrome. *Ophthalmol.* 1998;105:874-877.

[52] Parish HM, Somers VK. Obstructive sleep apnea and cardiovascular disease. *Mayo Clin. Proc.* 2004;79:1036-1046.

[53] Behbehani R, Mathews M, Sergott R, Savino P. Nonarteritic Anterior Ischemic Optic Neruopathy in Patients with Sleep Apnea While Being Treated with Continuous Positive Airway Pressure. *Am. J. Ophthalmol.* 2005;139:518-521.

Editor Contact Information

Mingwu Wang, MD, PhD

Department of Ophthalmology and Vision Science,
University of Arizona College of Medicine, AZ, US
Email:mwang@eyes.arizona.edu

Index

A

B

C

D

E

F

G

H

I

K

L

M

N

O

P

R

S

T

V